Introduction

My name is Karen, and I am 100 pounds overweight.

100 pounds ago, I sat in front of my camera, hit record, and made that statement. That's how this project started in March of 2012. Back then, I had been thinking about losing weight for quite a while. Like many people, I had some success with weight loss for a short period of time, and then I'd gain it back.

For the entirety of my adult life, I was obese. Even though I enjoyed sports, I instead busied myself with other things, and didn't stay fit or develop sustainable, healthy habits. The cycle of losing weight and gaining it back was endless. I felt hopeless, like a failure, like another statistic. Things eventually caught up to me, and I found my life had gotten to a point where I'd have to do something about it. Emotional and physical stress were wreaking havoc on my body. My mind was a mess. The decisions I was making, relationships I was in and my environment were toxic. I was miserable. I was punishing myself and allowing myself to be abused by others. I *let* it happen; I routinely associated love with abuse. This had been a common theme in my life: the relationships I had with family and loved ones, my romantic relationships, my behavior with food, alcohol, drugs, sex, work, video games...anything I loved, I'd do or use it to excess. It always ended badly, and I continued to hurt myself and let others hurt me.

Change happens when we need it, not when we're ready for it. When I finally accepted that my life needed a makeover, I sure wasn't ready, but I knew it had to happen. It was time to get very uncomfortable. It was time to do something very challenging.

When this started, I weighed 257 pounds, and wanted to lose 100 pounds. At five feet six inches tall, I felt that 157 pounds would be an ideal, healthy weight for my shape and height.

1

My first action was writing "100 reasons to lose 100 pounds" in big bold letters on top of a sheet of paper. I tore that sheet of paper out of my notebook, wrote the number 1 followed by the first reason, and I kept that sheet of paper with me, adding more reasons as they came to mind. The first few reasons came pretty easily. The next few came with some time. The remaining reasons took a bit longer, and then eventually, I had several sheets of paper with 100 reasons total.

Some of my reasons are pretty obvious – health, happiness and well-being. Some of them are interest-based, like sports, wearing costumes, and improving endurance. There are several reasons that are silly, even laughable – you'll see! There are also reasons that were inspired by deep hurts, like addiction, family drama, relationships, and the stresses of work and school.

My plan was to shoot 100 videos, each discussing a reason why I wanted to lose 100 pounds. I hoped that I would lose the 100 pounds and document the process with 100 videos, one for each pound lost.

I did it. I lost 100 pounds, and I shot 100 videos (they are linked in each reason of this book).

Now that I'm on the other end, I can look back and say that it's been an amazing ride! Any time we do something difficult and succeed, there's a great story that goes with it. The whole point of having experiences is to relate to others by sharing our successes and stories.

I hope my story gives hope, inspiration, and courage to anyone struggling with body image, self-worth, excess tendencies, addiction, sexual orientation, anger, mental illness, or any of the other issues that make us feel horribly. There IS hope. There IS support. There IS love out there, and there are ways to spark it and keep it roaring within.

It's all about love; how to find it in ourselves, around us in others, and in everything we see and do. It's not easy to change our lifestyle and habits, but, it's definitely worth it! The hard work pays off. It's a struggle, and good habits make it doable.

Weight loss had always seemed like a helpless, losing battle, and now that I've sustained a healthy lifestyle, I can happily say that it works! Over time, even with mistakes, we can rise from each fall, and we learn from every experience, good and bad. Life gives us lessons and blessings. They're all conducive to our personal growth.

Change happens in moments, one at a time. Those moments all add up!

It's my hope and dream to use my story to encourage, inspire, and motivate anyone struggling to find that light within and realize that you CAN do this!

Wishing you love, prosperity, success, and abundance, now and always!

From my heart to yours,
Karen Petersen

Preface

Do you struggle with excess tendencies? Do you have a troublesome relationship with food, exercise, alcohol, drugs, family, work, anger, stress, anxiety, intimacy, sexuality, and a host of other things?

Do you want to create habits to change your life for the better?

This book was written to give an honest, from-the-gut-account of a transition into a healthy lifestyle. My journey – changing my life and documenting it on video and in this book – required humility, honesty, and a willingness to make mistakes, learn from them, to be accountable, and to make difficult choices every day, moment to moment. My intention has always been to be open and sincere about my struggles as well as my triumphs. I made many mistakes. Sometimes I still do! However, I also celebrate victories. These go hand-in-hand; the victories are worthy of celebration *because* of the struggles it took to get there.

When I recorded the videos for the series, I did my best to note the date I recorded the video as well as my weight that day. Some of the videos are missing all of the specifics; however, they all have a reason from the original list of 100 Reasons to Lose 100 Pounds.

Through my experience, I found some of the reasons applicable after I hit my goal. As I've said before, I also discovered that some of them turned out differently than I had expected. I also discovered new reasons to *stay* healthy. For me, that just goes to show that there can often be a vast difference between what we want and what we need. I needed to get healthy, and it's my hope and dream to help reduce the obesity rate in our country and worldwide, to save lives, to spread hope and encouragement to people who have been neglected, abused, and bullied, and to help cut down on preventative illness. If my good health turned out to be the ONLY outcome of this project, then that is reason enough to keep going.

The biggest lesson I've gotten from losing 100 pounds and staying fit and healthy was that the journey is more important than the goal, because what we learn in the journey keeps the goal sustainable. After all, the work doesn't end when we reach our goal. For me, hitting my goal was just the beginning!

Every day I face the same challenges that I've always had. The difference now is that I have habits to help me make better decisions and to live a prosperous, content, spiritual, and healthy life. Instead of focus on maintaining a healthy lifestyle forever, I personally find it best to just focus on today. If I can make good choices today, then I've honored my goal and my journey. Tomorrow is another day. Today, this moment, being in the present is what gets me through.

Every day presents additional opportunities to lean, to grow, and to share our blessings and lessons with others. Every day is a blessing, and we will always find a lesson. Stay willing, stay committed, and document the process to remember what it was like, and to celebrate all the successes!

At the end of each reason in this book, there are some questions, assignments, activities or challenges. You may complete as many as you'd like. I suggest keeping a journal (a notebook works great!) to chronicle your own journey, and to address these questions. You can even start your own list of reasons! Remember to take it easy on yourself, and go at your own pace. After all, I'm not grading you and I'm certainly not judging you! If you can manage one reason a day and the corresponding challenge, that's wonderful! If that's too difficult, then do the best you can with the time you have. This is a journey, and an investment. Do what you can, when you can. As long as you're taking some time out for yourself every day and doing your very best, then you're already heading in an amazing direction!

We are in this together. You can do this. It CAN be done. It HAS been done!

Are you ready to change your life for the better? I'd LOVE to hear about your journey into wellness! I run a group called the Army of 100. Our group is meant to support and encourage people, and we've seen people in our world-wide group do amazing things! Join us, and be the next Smashing Success Story!

All of the links to each reason, each video for the reason, and the resources mentioned in this book can be found at http://mindheartswole.com/100reasonstolose100pounds/

100 Tips for Developing a Healthy Lifestyle

1. Compile a list of why you want to embark on a healthy lifestyle
2. Plan for solid rest
3. Develop a sleep schedule
4. There is only one Monday per week, and there are six other days. Why wait until Monday when you can start today? Start at any time. You can start your next meal. Start right now. Start with one simple habit and build on from there
5. Start a workout routine by doing something you enjoy for just FIVE minutes, three days a week. Build on that and work up to 10 minutes three days a week, then keep adding on five minutes per week until you hit 20 minutes of exercise for three days a week. Add more gradually. The point is to whet the appetite; starting with 30 minutes of exercise can be overwhelming, and 5 minutes is totally do-able! Take it easy on yourself. Set small, manageable, and realistic goals.
6. Remove the word "can't" from your vocabulary. Every time you feel like saying you can't, say "I CAN!" The result? You WILL!
7. No more complaining. Instead, come up with an action step to take to remedy the complaint. If nothing comes to mind, write it down, put it in a jar, and when the jar gets full, burn all the notes. Major catharsis!
8. Proper planning produces results! Plan your meals, and if you must eat out, know what is available before you order. Avoid impulsively purchased meals! When we plan properly, we're optimizing our time to focus on what we're good at and what's worth our time. Plan and prepare your meals in advance to spend more of your time where you can be a genius, doing what you do best, and doing what you LOVE to do!
9. Practice daily gratitude. This helps us shift our mindset from how things "should" be to appreciating everything that we have.
10. Tell yourself "I want to do this" instead of "I have to do this" whenever facing a challenge. That shift will work wonders!
11. Plan at least one rest/active recovery day. This doesn't mean lounging around all day; you can take a quiet, slow, meditative walk or practice restorative yoga. Give your body rest, but

avoid getting *too* restful.

12. Focus on daily goals and tasks. Instead of looking at the HUGE intimidating big picture, just focus on what can be done today. Habits are built over time and not established immediately. Pick one thing to start with.

13. Anything that sounds too good to be true very likely is. There is no easy way. The hard work is worth it, and it's done in moments, one at a time. Enjoy the journey instead of fixate on the destination!

14. Write an inspirational phrase on your mirror and say it daily. Some examples are:
"I'm worth it."
"We are as good as our greatest day, even if we have not had it yet."
"I'm a healthy and strong woman (or man)."
"I am absolutely fabulous!"
"Look how far I've come!"
"I've survived everything so far, I can now thrive."
Get creative and come up with some of your own!

15. Write your goals or type them up and print them. Hang them in places you'll see them regularly.

16. Buy an outfit a few sizes smaller than your current size. Only a few sizes. Try it on after a few months. Once it fits, wear it proudly, and then buy another outfit a few sizes smaller. Do this routinely, a few sizes at a time, until you can buy an outfit in your goal size.

17. Break things down into simple tasks. Instead of dreading a workout, just put on your workout clothes. Then, stretch. Then, start warming up, get yourself through each moment by staying present and go through each motion, one by one.

18. Set yourself up for success by having your workout clothes set out the night before, or even sleeping in them. Setting the stage is as important as walking on it.

19. Take deep breaths when stressed. Avoid reacting angrily. Those two seconds will change your life (I promise)!

20. Growth happens outside the comfort zone. When we lift weights, we build muscle by doing one or two repetitions past what we think we're capable of. These are magic moments. The

same thing happens when we rise to challenges.

21. Our bodies are machines, and way more evolved than our highly intelligent brains. Our bodies are more capable than our minds believe them to be. The limits in our brains are just the ego, wanting us to feel badly for ourselves, wanting us to feel significant because of the struggle. Meanwhile, your body grows *in spite* of the struggle. Your body grows *because* of the struggle. This is how we are conditioned, and this is how we have evolved.

22. Explore different workouts, group fitness classes, and all different types of sports and workouts. Take on a new hobby, like roller skating, dancing, and swimming. Mix things up as you go. Add variety to your routine. Explore. It will keep your curious, and it will engage your body in new and different ways!

23. Add one good habit at a time after you've mastered a new habit. By adding just one at a time, it becomes sustainable and you can build on from there. Give yourself at least a whole week of success with a new positive habit before adding another. Aim for one new healthy habit per month.

24. Give yourself lots of time. We hear the saccharine stories about "overnight success," but that is a complete and utter facade. The sensation was overnight; the success was the result of a lot of hard work, built over time. Even people who have had a lot of luck had a lot of tough breaks along the way. The good breaks are rare, and the tough times are plenty. That is why we celebrate the victories, and mourn the losses.

25. Choose to be a victor instead of a victim. Lots of things happen. When we shift our mentality into seeing it as an opportunity instead of a tragedy, we can then come up with solutions to deal with it. If we keep eating, drinking, and drugging our way through a pain, we can never really feel it and thus we cannot heal it. Feel. Then heal.

26. Think about what you can do and what you're capable of. Mobility issues, injuries, and certain limitations are not a handicap or a crutch; they present opportunities. You can still get fit and lose weight without full and comprehensive use of your body. There are plenty of athletes that are missing limbs,

have health issues, and have plenty of challenges. Instead of feeling victimized by their situation, they've used it as an opportunity to grow. Make a list of all the things that you can do, as opposed to fixate on what you can't do. Fitness is also matter of mindset.

27. Open your heart, allow yourself to be vulnerable. You don't have to tough your way through it. It takes more strength and courage to allow yourself to be vulnerable than it does to build up a wall. Strength is having the integrity to allow yourself to feel bad things.

28. Understand that good far outweighs the bad, and by opening ourselves up to better opportunities, we're able to walk away from the things that hurt us. Love doesn't hurt. Hurtful people hurt. Don't confuse codependency with love.

29. Make the right choice instead of the easy choice.

30. Put yourself as your priority. When you take care of yourself, everything else takes care of itself. Prioritize tasks. Make your health, wellness and fitness your priority.

31. Plan your day. Planning reduces stress because you're in charge and not merely reacting. Develop a schedule, plan your meals and workouts, and stick to your plan. Leave some room for the unexpected. Stay focused. Freedom comes from doing what you need to first, freeing time to do what you want to do later.

32. Dance, regardless of whether you're being watched, alone, or with others. It doesn't matter how it looks. Just have fun!

33. Throughout your day, breathe deeply and stretch often. Set timers on your phone to remind yourself (every hour or so).

34. Allow time for breaks in your busy/work times. Schedule breaks to breathe, go to the bathroom, refill your water, get fresh air, and so forth. Move a lot. It'll keep your body happy and your brain fresh!

35. Ask for help when you need it. Don't be shy. You've always got help available if you ask. Sometimes you may need to be persistent. Keep going!

36. Try a gym, fitness center and/or yoga studio before committing to a membership. Many have a buddy pass, guest pass or first class free option. Shop around. Go for a fitness center with a friendly and helpful staff, group fitness classes, accessible

hours, plenty of variety, and fewer frills (the less stuff – like juice bars-- the better the value for you). Go somewhere you feel comfortable. Don't get sold or pressured into a membership. Try it out. Try LOTS of them out until you find your fit!

37. Evaluate your goals weekly, and adjust as needed to keep them attainable and measurable. This will encourage you to stay on track!

38. Believe in yourself. It's a very simple concept, and even if it is a challenge to live it out, remind yourself that you *can* do it.

39. Replace bad habits (overeating, skipping workouts) with new, healthy habits. For instance, when you feel stressed, take ten deep, cleansing breaths. When bored, take a break and walk stairs. Read a book for a few minutes. Keep your mind busy.

40. Give yourself pep talks every time you look in the mirror. Admire your assets. Love your body as it is.

41. Document your journey. Keep a journal. Shoot video. Take pictures.

42. Do your measurements every few months and note the changes. Weighing in can be a bit deceiving when we're losing fat and building muscle, and measurements are a great way to mark progress!

43. The little things add up, so soak them up and enjoy EVERY positive step you're taking!

44. Don't sweat the small stuff. It really is just that – small stuff. By doing this, you'll ultimately see that all the things we worry about are just small, temporary annoyances.

45. Make a list of healthy foods you enjoy. Focus on what you like and what you can have, instead of what you "shouldn't" have.

46. Give yourself some space and allowance for a cheat meal once to three times a week (if you have three cheat meals, have them on separate, non-consecutive days). Keep portions in moderation. We tend to go all-out on both ends of the spectrum (too "healthy"/restrictive, and then overly excessive). The "secret" to sustainable healthy living is to find balance! Think in terms of moderation, instead of elimination. You don't have to give up your favorite things. Just do them more sensibly. For instance, you can have pizza, wings, burgers, fries, and ice cream. You can have these things, just not all in one sitting, or

in one day! Leave room for cheat meals, and an occasional cheat day. Allow yourself to enjoy things that you regularly enjoy. By doing so in moderation, it will prevent the bad habit of over indulging.

47. A personal favorite trick – eat the biggest meal in the middle of the day. This gives your body the rest of the day to burn.

48. Eat your carbohydrates, especially earlier in your day! Forget crash-and-burn diets! NO DIETS! Eat reasonably. Our bodies need proteins, fats AND carbohydrates!

49. Eat lots of fruits and vegetables. When it comes to vegetables, eat as MANY as you'd like, especially leafy greens! Eat sweet potatoes and legumes (beans) in moderation.

50. For supper, eat lean proteins and vegetables. If you must have carbohydrates (for instance, if you're eating supper after a workout), make those carbohydrates simple, like vegetables and sweet potatoes (instead of white potatoes, pasta, rice, beans and sugary foods). Just watch your portions.

51. Limit alcohol consumption. Avoid drinking your calories. Personally I suggest eliminating alcohol altogether. Find what works best for you. If you cannot cut it out totally, limit yourself to one to two drinks maximum per week. Do this on the day before your rest day. Even one alcoholic drink will affect your workouts – guaranteed!

52. Eat slowly. Take small bites. Eat mindfully. Pray between fork/spoonfuls. Honor each meal. This is how we fuel our bodies. It's an act of self-love and maintenance. If we've abused food in the past, this is a great time to change how we view, consume, and think about food. Food is a necessity. Let's stop resenting it and develop better attitudes and habits with food.

53. It's much easier to resist temptation when there are only healthy food options in the house. Remove all unhealthy and trigger foods from the pantry, refrigerator and freezer. Stock only healthy options.

54. When obsessing about a specific food, question yourself: Is it available in single-serving? Can I split it with someone? Why am I craving this?

55. Slowly wean yourself off of sugary sweets and drinks. Don't sweat eliminating things completely. Switch from sodas to diet

sodas if you must, preferably sparkling water with natural flavoring added, or to flavored non-carbonated water.

56. Keep your mouth busy by chewing gum, coffee stirrers or straws. Quite often the oral fixation is a psychological addiction.

57. Try all kinds of healthy recipes. Cut the recipe as needed, depending on how many people you're serving. If it's a 6-serving recipe and you're cooking for yourself, cut the recipe in half. Once you've made your plate, put the remaining two portions into two containers for meals later in the week!

58. Eat smaller portions of your favorite foods. Focus on moderation instead of total elimination.

59. Add healthy foods into your diet. Add variety by trying different fruits and vegetables.

60. Reduce portions and eat more often. Eat three small meals, with two to three snacks, instead of two or three big meals per day.

61. Eat breakfast. This bears repeating - eat breakfast. I'll repeat it again. Eat. Breakfast.

62. Stay away from supplements. Supplements are a subsidiary of the diet industry, which is a multi-billion-dollar industry with a 95% failure rate. Avoid sensation, and focus on changing your lifestyle. There is no quick fix. Supplements are pushed on desperate people like drugs are pushed onto addicts. Sure, they give you a lot of stuff for free at first, but that is how they draw you in.

63. Avoid getting into any weight loss products, and especially avoid selling these products. Stay away from expensive wraps, pills, meal replacement supplements, energy products and other non-regulated items. Just eat healthy, exercise, and develop a mindfulness routine (like prayer and meditation).

64. If you really want to spend the money on health products, switch over to organic produce.

65. Think about textures, and replace go-to craving foods with healthier options. For instance, if you like crunchy things like chips, get lots of raw veggies, like carrots. Carrots are very healthy, inexpensive, & a great grab-and-go type food. Buy a bunch of carrots, peel them, and now you have a snack anytime. It's always better to overindulge in carrots instead of a bag of

potato chips!

66. Learn to roast vegetables - it's very simple. Chop them up, mix with a bit of olive oil, salt and pepper. Roast them 425 Fahrenheit for at least 30 minutes, stirring and checking on them every 20 minutes or so until they are beautifully browned. Roasted vegetable are delicious, a great source of nutrients, and a guilt-free healthy meal!

67. If you tend to eat big portions, start adding healthy, homemade soups into your meal plans. Add lots of vegetables.

68. Salads are another great way to eat a lot of food without taking in excessive calories. Fill them with fresh vegetables and dress them simply with lemon juice or portioned homemade dressings.

69. End your meal with a big hot mug of tea. Herbal tea is a great way end of the evening.

70. Food is fuel, so treat your body like a high-performance machine. Feed yourself well, often, and plenty!

71. Read labels carefully. Often "natural" can be deceiving. Watch out for added sugars!

72. Avoid sugar-free and fat-free substitutes. Often sugar-free substitutes have added fat, and fat-free substitutes have added sugar.

73. Choose more foods with no labels and a short shelf-life: fresh produce, lean meats, and unprocessed whole foods.

74. Food that can be prepared in bulk, portioned into containers, and frozen are a great way to optimize your time and resources. Find loads of recipes that are healthy, simple, and appealing to you. Start with what you're familiar with and get curious.

75. Shop for in-season, local produce whenever possible. This will save you money and you'll get the best there is when produce is at its peak!

76. Research sale items, seasonal items and specials, and design your menu and meal plans around what's available to save money.

77. Log your meals and your moods each time you eat. This will help you notice patterns – especially cravings associated with moods!

78. Understand hunger versus boredom. Your mood, activity level

and logs will help you notice this.

79. To understand what hunger feels like, have a meal in front of you, push it away, and think about eating it. Imagine the first bite. Meditate on this for several moments, and then eat. Then, leave the last bite on the plate. That will give good perspective!

80. Remove trigger foods from your home. If you want a treat or are planning a cheat meal, go out and get it, and don't stock it in the house!

81. Surround yourself with people and things that inspire you. If something (or someone) is dragging you down, evaluate how important it is and how it contributes to your wellness. Sometimes, things have to go, and that's okay. Let them go.

82. Read daily inspiration! Fill your mind with motivational and encouraging words, pictures and phrases!

83. Tell your family and friends about your journey into a healthy lifestyle and ask for their support. Often our spouses, significant others, close family and friends may offer temptations and say things like, "you're great the way you are" (and you certainly are). They are trying to be supportive. Thank them for loving you. However, if this seems like sabotage, it may very well be. Politely decline any temptations that may cause you to over-indulge.

84. Listen to upbeat music, whether you are working out, planning your playlist for the next workout, or just doing things around the house! Listen to energizing music when you want to be energized – don't just save it for your workouts.

85. Laugh often. Read funny stories. Look up cat videos online. Read the comics. Find plenty of reasons to smile!

86. Develop a buddy system. Encourage others to join you in your quest. Call these people when things are challenging or when you have great news, or to lend an ear when they need to talk. We get outside of ourselves by finding the company of others. Curiosity cures loneliness.

87. Find mentors. Choose successful who have what you want. Offer to help them, and seek people who are willing to help you.

88. Follow social media of people you admire. Surround yourself with positive influence.

89. Limit contact with people who drain you, complain incessantly, and have horrible habits. This doesn't make them "bad people," it just makes them bad influences.
90. Ask the right questions to the right people. For instance, speak with a nutrition advisor about meal plans. Ask a personal trainer about a fitness plan. Go to the right people for the appropriate things.
91. When you meet people who have what you want, ask them lots of questions. Listen to their answers intently. Don't compare, complain, and rationalize why you "can't" (remember - we eliminated that word) to them! They have their own journey and you have yours. Just as they're great and successful at something, you are great and successful at something.
92. Try different mobile applications, websites and tools to help you in your journey. Some great ones are: Sparkpeople, My Fitness Pal, Endomondo, and WOD Box. Ask around and try a bunch!
93. Talk among your friends and family, and recruit them in your journey! Create a group, host dinners, crafting parties, group meetings and discussions! Plan meals together, have a group cooking day – crock pot swaps are great! Everyone brings a crock pot and ingredients, cooks their respective meal and when they're done, everyone takes home a variety of meals from everyone who participated!
94. Plan your work, and work your plan. Stick with it. Leave room for rest, recovery, and rewards!
95. Treat yourself with rewards for hitting milestones! The only rule here – do not use food as a reward.
96. Experiences make for GREAT rewards!
97. Massages are a great reward!
98. Trips and vacations are another awesome reward!
99. Buying a new piece of fitness equipment is an excellent reward – a bicycle, free weights, a yoga mat and new sneakers are wonderful!
100. Print this list and add more ideas as you think of them!

<u>100 Reasons To Lose 100 Pounds</u>
<u>A Smashing Transformation in Mind, Body and Spirit</u>

by Karen Petersen

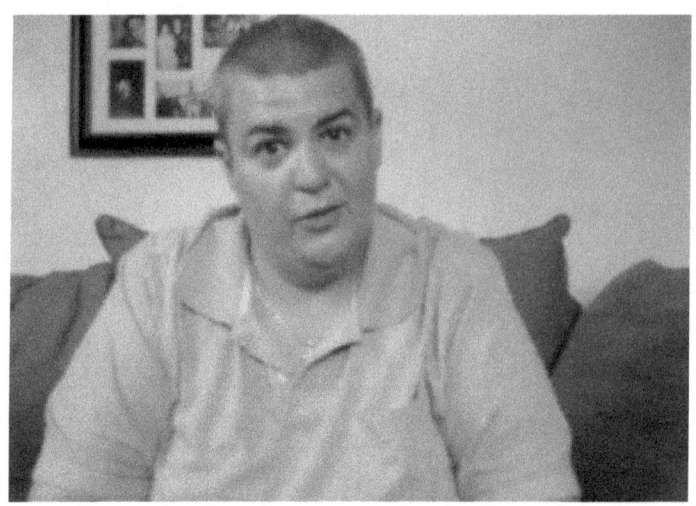

Reason #1: <u>To heal and recover, physically and emotionally</u>
Recorded on March 3, 2012
Weight: 257 pounds

When I started this series, all I had was an idea, the desire, and a list of 100 Reasons to Lose 100 pounds of excess body fat. At 257 pounds, losing 100 pounds of fat would put me at a healthy weight for my height and build.

On paper, I had gotten away with poor health for a while. Eventually, I wasn't getting away with it any longer. Stress, bad relationships, my job, and a lack of exercise combined with eating too much food (and unhealthy food) took its toll, and I realized that I wasn't taking care of myself. That needed to change.

Though I still struggled with accepting myself as a person (let alone a heavyset person), overall, I knew that I have a good soul and that I deserved to be loved, especially by myself. I wanted to let my huge, brilliant, inner light shine, and yet I knew the excess fat was holding me back from truly moving forward to where I wanted to be in my life.

I knew I wanted to lose the weight, and as hard as it would be and as long as it would take, it had to start somewhere.

Healing emotionally, I knew, would also be a huge building block to improving my health. For a long time, I was very angry. Anxiety had always been a huge part of my story, and I was living with constant stress. Life had presented me with bigger challenges and eventually, anger, frustration and anxiety started causing me physical issues. I decided that managing stress (especially my lifestyle) would be the key to get me healthy again. This time, I knew that if I wanted to feel well and have my energy back, I had to change my habits.

Physical movement has always been something I enjoy, and I can spend hours working out, doing outdoor tasks and generally getting hot and sweaty. The biggest problem for me has always been how I eat and what I eat. Unfortunately, it takes longer to work off excess calories than it does to ingest them. Ten minutes of bad food choices can make an hour-long workout go down the drain. Once I got a good handle on my bad habits, the physical health benefits would naturally follow.

With all this in mind and armed with awareness, motivation, and 99 more reasons, this was the moment that I had enough and was ready for something better. I was ready to take ownership of how I allowed myself to be treated, especially by myself.

So, I got out my digital camera and started recording, without a clue about how I was going to do it. I just knew that I wanted to, and that I was capable of it.

This is the first reason that I recorded, and every time I see a screen shot or watch it again, I'm so damn proud of myself for doing this. Can I believe that was me? Hell yeah I can! I still see that woman, I still think some of those thoughts, and sometimes, I still feel sadness like I did back then. However, now my lifestyle has adjusted, and so have my habits. The thoughts don't linger the same way because I am taking good care of myself.

We all have things we want to do to improve our lives, and the biggest step is to take the first step. Talking and thinking only go so far. Action gets things done.

It took me a long time to do it, and it's going to take a lifetime to keep going. It's worth the effort. It's worth doing it because I choose to. I want to!

Reason #1 is huge because it's when I finally understood that I have to take care of myself. I needed to focus on me. I was the only one that could do it.

The first step can be the hardest, and so many of us talk about it. Very few follow through. Even fewer keep going. It's those who persist who are successful.

I chose to give it hell!

I *still* do!

Questions:
How do you feel now?
How do you want to feel?
Is your lifestyle affecting your health?

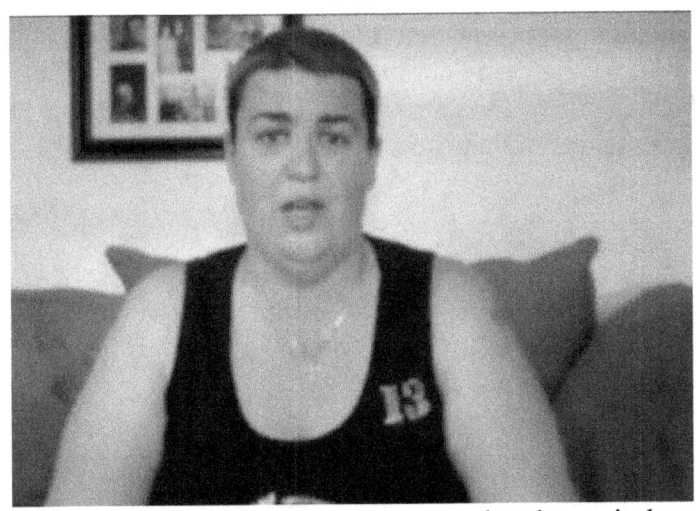

Reason #2: <u>So I can find peace and a clear mind</u>
Recorded on April 17, 2012
Weight: 249 pounds

I've read that stressing an event is worse than the stress of the event itself, so I wanted to stop thinking the same, repetitive, damaging thoughts. Finding clarity had always been an issue for me, so I wanted to focus on acceptance and gratitude.

Things that have also helped me stay calm along the journey (and after as well):

1. Make good nutritional choices – they affect mood, overall outlook, sleep patterns and curb cravings
2. Don't push too hard – going at a steady pace keeps things sustainable
3. Keep realistic goals – expecting too much too soon only leads to disappointment and discouragement

Using these things, I started building good habits, and once I found consistency, I'd add more things, one at a time. I went from eating about once or twice a day (in vast portions and drinking sodas and coffee all day) to eating three to five smaller meals throughout the day.

My soda consumption went from three to five a day down to one a day, then one a week, and then I cut them out totally. Coffee was eliminated as well. Portion control was also becoming a habit, and I was allowing myself an occasional indulgence. I was finding balance.

From the video for Reason #2:
Keeping calm and finding peace and a clear mind is a day by day, one day at a time process, just like this weight loss is. I'm hoping as I continue to be successful, it'll affect other components of my life, too. Here's to the next one, one day at a time.

It was, it has been, and I fully acknowledge that it will always be.

It's worth it!

Activity:
Read this, and then close your eyes and do the activity.
Imagine something that upsets you, stresses you out, and frustrates you. See this clearly in your mind. Take a deep breath in, and imagine putting that situation into a balloon. Fill the balloon in your mind, and as you exhale, imagine that balloon has been released. Take nine more breaths by slowly inhaling, imagining peace, love and light filling you. With each exhale, feel relief; accept it and receive it. When you finish the tenth breath, take one more deep breath in, eyes open, mind at ease, and exhale, feeling the release of whatever you've been holding onto. Let the positive energy replace that stress. Do this every time you feel stressed out about something. If you don't have time for ten breaths, take at least five.

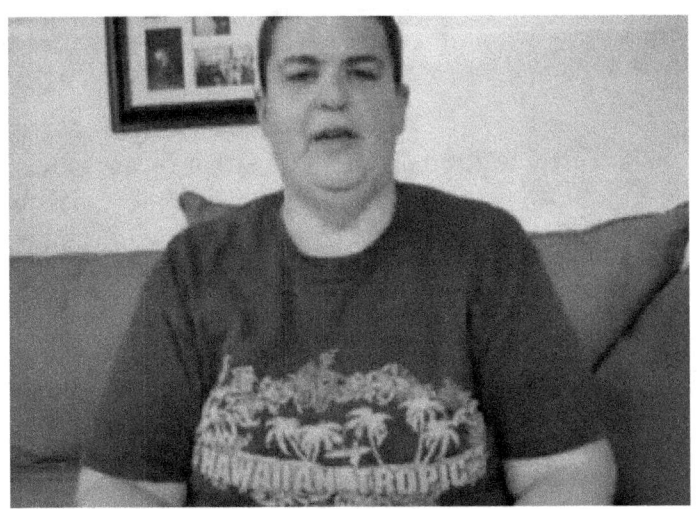

Reason #3: <u>To look and feel great</u>
Recorded on April 24, 2012

When we see images promoting weight loss, diets, and gyms, we see fit, beautiful, ideal and sculpted people talking about how we can do it, too. That image tricks us into thinking we can look like that, and it engenders an idea that there is a certain *look* associated with health.

I bought into the idea that looks are an indication of overall well-being. I thought losing weight would make me look a certain way. Now I know that's definitely not the case. I see the merits of this reason, and I also know why I originally came up with it.

The reasons were written and the series was recorded as I was making a big transition in my life – particularly, after a break-up. I wanted to feel empowered, so I was fixated on looking hot so I could look and feel desirable. Now that I've done it, that attention, to be forthright, makes me super skeptical.

We all want people to be how we idealize them to be, and good-looking people are, on the whole, well-liked and given extra passes by society. Good-looking folks tend to get more of the things we desire – sex, power, getting away with things and given many, many extra chances. I wanted to get in on that.

Looking good was for my ego, but admitting that I want to feel great was for my soul. I wanted to feel healthy in mind, body and spirit. That happens not by "losing weight", but by changing my *life* and my *thoughts.*

Now people tell me "you look so much better," and ask me "who was that girl"?

I am and have always been the same person, so "looking good" now doesn't necessarily make me "feel great". I look good because I feel good, and I feel good because I take good care of myself!

When I shot Reason #3, I had just finished watching Fat, Sick, and Nearly Dead, and I wanted to follow Joe Cross's 10-day juice cleanse.

This was another endeavor that sounded so much better than the reality of it!

About the juice cleanse: To put it bluntly, I hated it! I did it for ten days total and felt tired, irritable, and SO hungry ALL the time! I needed at least ten hours of sleep per night, and my workouts were limited to short walks. I even bulked up my juices with banana, avocado and whole mangoes, and still didn't feel energized. It was on the eighth day out of ten that I finally started getting my energy back. In those ten days, I lost a LOT of weight. A LOT. Like 14 pounds!

After I got back on solid food, I gained some of it back immediately, and the rest of it compounded shortly after.

In short, it was good because it taught me about moderation and appreciating food. While I was on the fast, I was very dedicated and stuck with it. It helped me realize that when I set a goal, I see it through. It was bad for sustainability, satisfaction, feeling full (which, for me, is a necessary component to stick with a nutrition plan), and especially for my energy. The film said it would take about four days for the mood and energy to re-calibrate. For me, it took twice that time.

Since the cleanse, I have not gone on another juice cleanse, and I really don't want to again!

I'm glad I tried it, and it taught me what actually works for me: regular exercise, staying calm, eating clean, and allowing some indulgence in moderation (portion control is key!).

Assignment:
Put on your favorite outfit, get dressed up, do your hair, put on perfume/cologne and then stand in front of the mirror. Admire how amazing you look. Own that look! Look yourself in the eyes and just soak it all in. Spoil yourself for the sake of spoiling yourself. Look good for *you*. When we dress up and feel good, we attract positive attention because it's shining from within! Tell yourself positive things about how you feel and how you look. Give yourself a wink and say something to yourself that you like hearing others say to you. Some examples are:
"Hey gorgeous!"
"You look beautiful!"
"Hello, stud!"
"You are glowing!"
"Wow, look at you owning that! Rock on!"

Grab your notebook/journal and write how you feel. Accept and love yourself now, in this moment. Appreciate how good you look and feel.

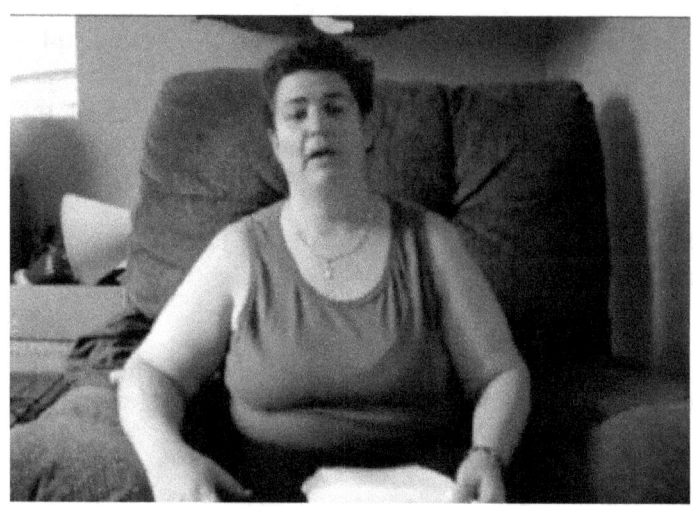

Reason #4 – <u>Because people will compliment me on my progress</u>
Recorded on July 31, 2012

Eating right, exercising, and getting enough sleep.
This is from the video for Reason 4. These are common knowledge.
We all know what we are *supposed* to do in order to be healthy.
Knowing and doing are very different.

When I recorded this reason, I had implemented strategies and was
getting compliments, and actually seeing the changes myself. Getting
compliments are great, but in all honesty, it didn't turn out the way I
expected it to.

Compliments were hard to accept. It was hard for me to allow all this
good energy into my life when, for so long, I neglected to allow it in. I
was fearful. My concept of love was always coupled with manipulation
and abuse. So, when complimented, I felt like someone *wanted
something from me.*

It's taken a long time for me to break out of my old thinking. Now, I
know that I control how I receive compliments. People may say kind
things for the sake of being kind. I can take it for what it is worth. That

has eased the burden of expectation – I don't expect anything when kindness is shared, and they don't expect anything in return.

Questions:
How do you feel when you compliment someone?
How does it feel when people say nice things to you?
Would you like to be treated kindly?
Do you think you deserve to be treated with love and respect? Why?

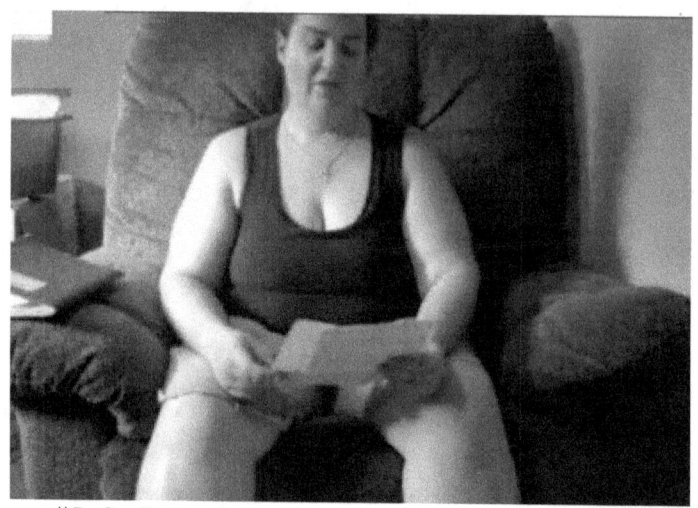

Reason #5: <u>So I can share my experience and encourage people</u>
Recorded on September 17, 2012
Weight: 237 pounds

When I started writing my list, I knew that sharing my experience with others was going to be a big component. By sharing what I was going through, I hoped to relate to others who have also struggled with obesity. I wanted to help proliferate healthy lifestyles.

It's important to share our own successes so that others can learn how to do it. Being honest, real, and sincere about the victories as well as the setbacks is great encouragement to people, because mistakes teach us lessons. Sharing enables others to learn from our mistakes, and shows that it's okay to mess up. Successful people make mistakes all the time! Life is never a straightforward path, and we learn to adapt.

Even today, I have struggles. Sometimes, a cheat meal turns into a cheat day and a cheat weekend. Instead of give up, berate myself, or go to extremes, I just get back to healthy eating, working out and eating the right portions of the right foods. Mistakes happen! It's what we do after that makes a huge difference.

Sharing is also important for me because it keeps me accountable. Documenting and speaking about my journey are constant reminders of where I've been, and doing so keeps me headed in the right direction.

While going through the experience I needed all the encouragement I could get. I still do! I've been successful because of the work others before me have shared, because of what I've read (I keep an updated list on my website here: http://mindheartswole.com/mind/), and by listening to the stories of people who have what I want, and have worked hard to get it. I learned from others before me, and I realized that my story will help others write their own!

Activity:
If you haven't already, take a picture of yourself, as your "before" image. Be your true self – no fake smiles, and no forced frowns. Just be real. Be in comfortable clothes, and allow yourself to be raw and authentic. Write down the day and time you've taken this picture, and print it out.

Go out and get a poster board, and put your picture on it. Write three key phrases on top, and make this your mantra (for instance, my three phrases are: moderation, loveable, acceptance. I'll say a mantra of, "I practice moderation in good nutrition, workouts, and work. I am loveable. I am accepted as I am"). Find images from magazines that appeal to you and are conducive to your goals. Pictures of healthy meals, fruits, salads, and snacks work great! Post these to your board. Leave spaces for in-progress pictures, and for noting the dates (and weights or measurements if you'd like). Have a big space reserved for your goal spot, and mark it. Have a path on your board leading to this spot. As you work toward your goal, fill the spaces with empowering, positive and uplifting things documenting your journey. Put your board in a highly visible area. Look at it every day. Say the mantra out loud every time you look at your board.

Share this activity with people and host a crafting day!

One of my visuals is my tracking board – this board represents my starting weight and each of the 100 pounds I wanted to lose to hit my goal weight. I still have it and it's a great reminder of where I've been, why I did this, and how I did it!

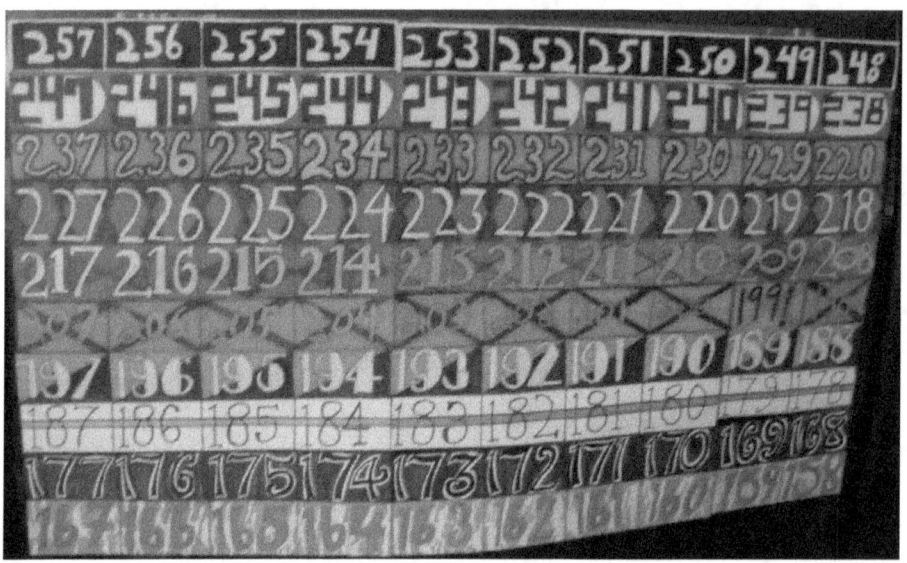

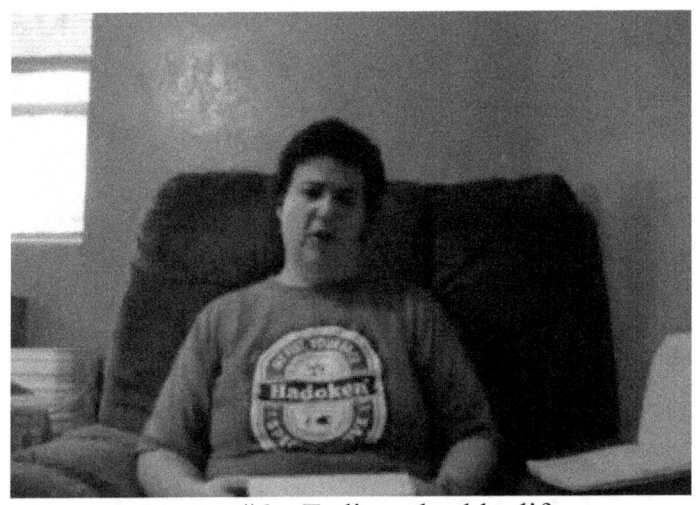

Reason #6 – <u>To live a healthy life</u>
Recorded in September 2012
Weight: 234 pounds

A healthy life is an integration of good habits in mind, body and spirit. By eating healthier foods in smart portions; moving my body; surrounding myself with motivational, inspirational and uplifting images and messages; and having a spiritual practice (praying and meditating regularly), I built habits that contribute to my overall well-being.

It happens in moments, every day. Little by little. There's no right time to start. There's only now.

From the video for this reason:
I had a realization and I was ready to make the commitment and build the habits…it really hit me that now is the time. I kept saying, 'okay, Monday…okay next Monday', but it really starts with today….one thing at a time.

Reviewing my journal at the time, I chose to write things I like about myself, and then I decided to share them in the video. Here's the list!

What I like about myself

I am: Brave, honest, smart, good, sincere, genuine, idealistic, loving, kind, successful, resourceful, respectable, funny, intelligent, cute, inspiring, bold, strong, insightful, loyal, trustworthy, and good-looking.

It's taken a LONG time to allow myself to see the good, the beauty, and the potential in me. Now I can go into any store and try on clothes right from the rack. I can keep up in group fitness classes. I can dine out without worrying about what other people think. I've got the courage, training and endurance to teach awesome fitness and yoga classes. Just like I'm writing this book to encourage people, I've also been leading online communities and sharing insight, encouragement and support for people who want and need confidence-boosters.

Feeling confident can still be a struggle at times, which is a reminder about why habits are so immensely important. Good habits inspire good action. I want to be healthy, happy, and feel at peace with myself.

It took a few months to find a fairly consistent rhythm, and it started with steps that became strides.

Once I found consistency with my nutrition and workouts, I found more and more relief physically. My stress levels dropped, and I was relied less on medication.

Assignment:

Grab your notebook and a pen. Take five deep breaths, eyes closed, and clear your mind. Once you've completed the breathing assignment, open your book and spend the next ten minutes writing down your assets. If you pause or can't think of anything, take more deep breaths, staying calm and clearing your mind, and write as soon as they come to you. Focus on your assets instead of your perceived defects. Write until the time is up, or you can't think of any more, and if you run out of time, keep writing! Leave plenty of space on this page or pages, and keep adding more as you think of them!

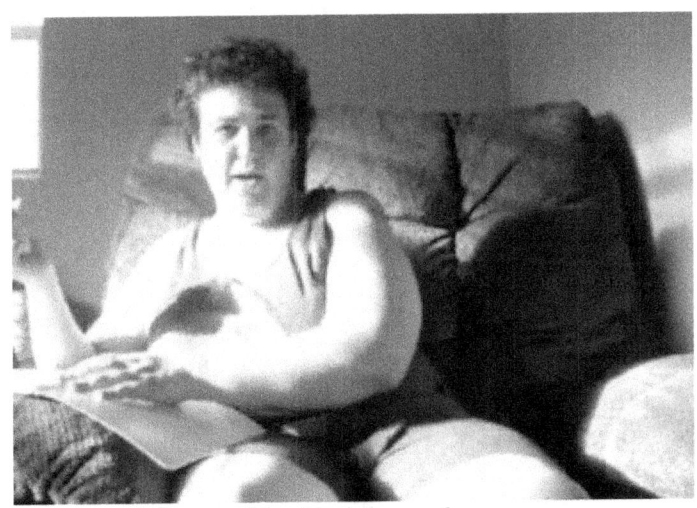

Reason #7 – <u>To take up less space</u>
Recorded on September 26, 2012

I heard a story about how someone was denied access to a theme park
ride because she was too large for the ride. As she exited the line, she
was ridiculed and laughed at. It broke my heart to hear that. No one
deserves that.

It's happened to me. I was in Las Vegas with a loved one, and we were
waiting in line for one of the rides on top of the Stratosphere. When we
got to the ride, I was unable to fit into the seat and had to get off the
ride. The person I was with went on without me. I was devastated.
After this person finished the ride, she asked me, "You want to check
out other rides that you're too fat for?"

In the past, there were several situations where proximity was very
uncomfortable. I was terrified on rides because I thought I would break
their safety devices. I hated flying because my elbows and side belly
would touch the person or people next to me. Sitting in movie theaters
was a massive pain in the ass.

Having a large frame also caused physical discomfort. When seated, I
leaned over a lot, often hunching my shoulders. It was difficult to sit

33

upright because my belly pulled me forward and pushed my arms further to the side.

I won't even begin to discuss how difficult it was to ride a bicycle (especially before I got the super wide padded seat). OUCH.

Now, I can spin, cycle, and sit comfortably in theaters, airplanes, cars – you name it. Dining out has been vastly improved, both physically and emotionally. I can fit into any seat, booth, and stool, and I don't feel like the lonely fat girl when I dine alone. Also, when dining out with friends, I no longer feel insecure about my meal options, whether I'm eating something healthy (which I now do by choice, instead of eating it because I felt like I was being judged), or if I'm having a cheat meal. When I have a healthy meal, I'm eating it because I want to eat healthy. When I have a cheat meal, I know I've earned it!

This reason and hearing about what others experience reminds me why I wanted to write this.

We're not alone. We're never alone. We all struggle. However, we can do something about it.

It's worth the work. Especially if you LOVE roller coasters like I do!

Questions:
Have you ever been taunted and/or turned away from anything because of your size?
Have you see this happen to another person?
How did that make you feel?
Did you want to do something about it?

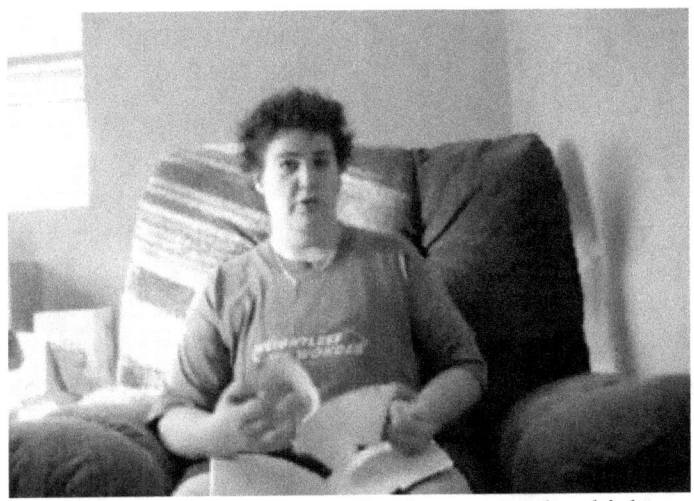

Reason #8 – <u>So I can not only play sports, but kick ass</u>
Recorded on: October 22, 2012
Weight: 228 pounds

When I started the list and got serious about losing excess fat, one of my intentions was to become a roller derby athlete. I had already met with a local team and started to become acquainted with some of the women who played. It was easy to get hooked immediately, especially after some of their best skaters assured me that they too had zero skating background.

Being a great athlete doesn't mean being the very best, it means being our own best. I knew that my personal best would come from getting into great shape. I still work on things off-skates to improve my skating and my overall fitness, such as core exercises and balance work to keep me strong and steady on my skates, and plyometric exercises to attack a big hill with ease. Yoga has been tremendously beneficial for my skating – both physically and mentally!

There is no comfort zone when it comes to training. In order to grow, we push past what we are comfortable with. It doesn't have to be a grueling experience –Growth is measured when we ask if we can keep going for a bit more. We grow when we push hard, feel like that's almost all we have, and then go a bit further. The best-trained athletes know how to tap into this extra push because they train for it. It's uncomfortable and taxing, but it is so worth the hard work and the effort.

Respect is given to (and earned by) the athlete who never gives up, and pushes his or her own limits. They may not have the most skill, but their drive is inspiring. Training for that is physical and mental. That kind of training is a lesson in letting the body go past what the mind believes it is capable of. It's trusting our bodies to grow past what feels comfortable, and letting the limiting thoughts in our head subside.

Those habits also touch other areas of our lives – and that's another reason to work toward our very best!

Assignment:
This is a visualization exercise.

Imagine you are in the arena of choice in your favorite type of event. Make it something that you're either good at, or something you want to do. Aim high. Make it one of your biggest dream activities. Imagine yourself as your "after": fit, toned, smiling and confident. Everything is in your favor. Let your imagination run wild. Imagine the most ideal circumstances, in the best environment, under the best conditions, and as the perfect person. Everything will go your way.

Take at least ten minutes and observe everything in this scenario. How amazing you are doing your thing. What smells surround you? Who is there? What is the outcome? Imagine how you feel. What does it feel like?

You may go as long as you'd like, so take at least ten minutes. Then, write a full description of what you were doing, and everything you can think of detailing the experience. Remember to imagine all of your senses, and describe how they were all affected. Include every detail. Go big!

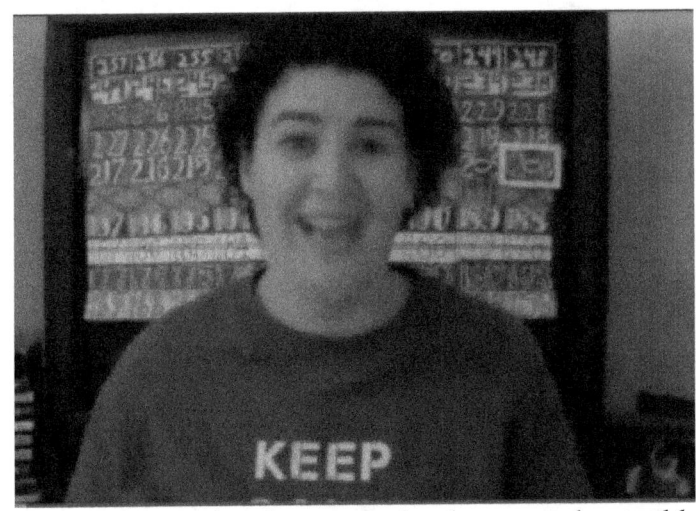

Reason #9 – <u>For sexual endurance and to be more pleasurable to my partner.</u>
Recorded on November 29, 2012
Weight: 208 pounds

Getting healthy, for me, also meant being very selective about who I share my time, my life, and my body with. This journey gave me more self-worth, and with that came the dichotomy of both wanting to share this body a lot, or to hold out for something valuable and substantial. In the process, I learned the latter is what I truly yearn for.

The way I see it, if I'm going to work this hard to get into great shape, hold out for someone special, and finally share myself with her, it better be worth the wait! It better be worth it for BOTH of us!

Also, since I've worked so hard to get to this point (and the next phase, and after that), that person will also have worked hard to get to me. It takes experience to recognize a familiar trait in another, and the same things I have to offer are what I would want in another. A part of that is to enjoy a healthy physical relationship!

I feel joyful, abundant and satisfied when my lover is satisfied. My pleasure in a physically intimate encounter comes from hearing, watching, and feeling my partner's reactions. There are so many ways

37

to please a lover – as many ways as there are lovers, and every lover has several ways she enjoys sex. It's an adventure discovering someone's needs and wants. This is a great place for me to toss in one of my favorite quotes about being gay: when I'm asked, "how do women have sex with each other?" my favorite response is, "the question isn't how we do it, the question is how do we stop?!" It's so spot-on, I love it. Since we don't have a one-shot ending, we can go on and on, for hours on end, til the sun rises and sets again. When I wrote this reason, I had already experienced that myself, so I could only imagine what was possible once I became fit!

Questions:
How do you feel when you see yourself nude?
If you could see yourself through your partner's (past or present) eyes, how do you see yourself?
How do you see your sex life improving? What would improve it?

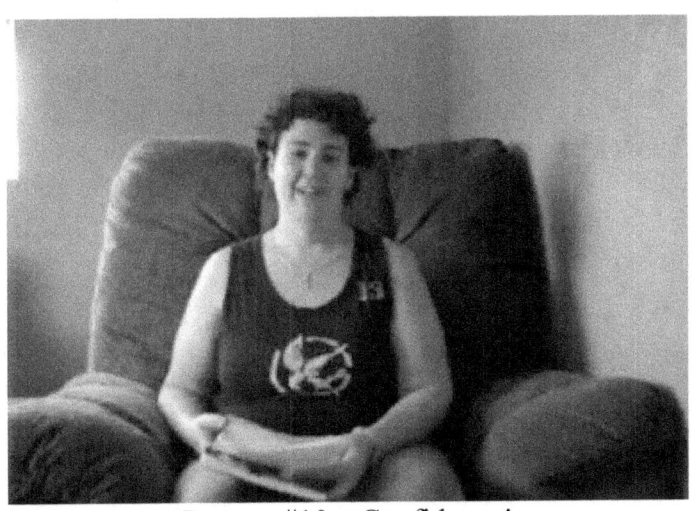

Reason #10 – Confidence!
Recorded on November 30, 2012
Weight: 207 pounds

How dare we be modest when we're capable of being great? Are we afraid of being mocked for being confident?

Being confident is VERY different from being self-centered, egotistical, competitive, or elitist. Very, very different indeed. Confidence acknowledges the rock star that we all are. It's an awareness of the results from all the work we've put in. Confidence doesn't compete, it collaborates, by sharing our success strategies with others, guiding and watching them become empowered, and cheering them on when they excel! Some people even surpass us, which is fantastic! When we can be happy for others, that shows that we're happy with ourselves and can admire another person without taking offense to their success. That's something that people with integrity can do – be confident, and be happy for other people, especially when they get what we have and want!

Confidence, for me, had to be earned. My whole life, I had allowed myself to be spoken down to. I felt like I was a piece of shit. My self-worth was so low; I allowed the opinions of others to penetrate my mind. I allowed physical abuse. I believed I deserved it.

No more of that! Now, I stand up for myself. Staying positive comes naturally. The more I push past the desire to speak negatively, the more positive things I attract. Showing up big (rising to the occasion with adult-pants on instead of diapers, so to speak) in difficult and intimidating situations has become routine for me. Now, when I want something, I go for it.

When I show my "before" pictures, which I LOVE, people ask me, "can you believe who that person is?" Of course I do. I'm still that person! The outside may look different, but the things that go on inside still exist. We can't change our past or the things that have shaped and molded us into the people that we are. It's actually those things that give us the strength to step it to the next level. We either fall from the pressure, or we rise with strength. Strength builds confidence! Every day, I am reminded how strong I really am.

Confidence comes from success. I gained mine when I got rid of a lot of negative influences that inspired my self-destructive behaviors. Now, I surround myself with uplifting people and images.

I love to look at old pictures and think about how far I've come! It's a great boost!

Assignment:
Call someone you admire, and tell them why you admire them. Point out something or things that they have done and ask them how they did it, and what the experience was like. Listen mindfully, without the need to interject, compare or complain. Keep asking questions. Thank that person for being in your life, and ask if you could meet him or her for lunch, your treat. Set a day and follow up with that person and hear what he or she has to say.

It takes courage and confidence to listen to someone without taking his or her success personally. Do this with someone who is successful, and learn from their example!

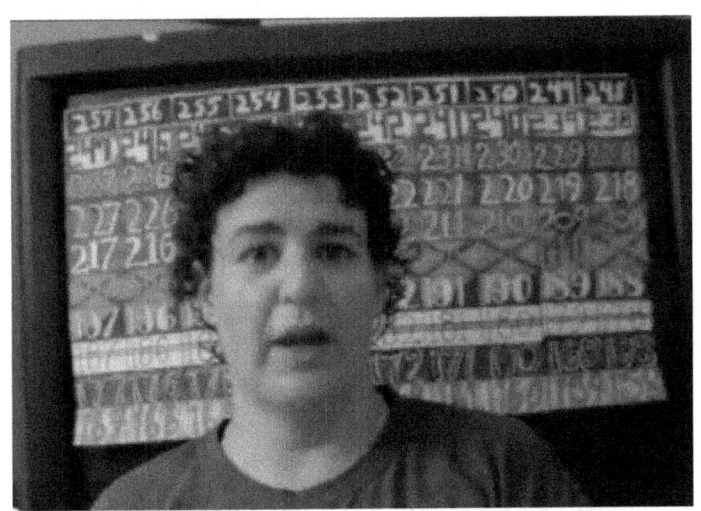

Reason #11 – <u>To understand myself better</u>
Recorded on December 3, 2012

From the video for this reason:
It's when we go through our hardest times that we become the strongest...there is nothing that can defeat me...I don't quit, I don't give up. There's one thing that's more powerful than any force, any thing, or any entity that is living, breathing and existing on this planet, and that's the power of the human will. I don't know about you, but I have the power to succeed...I know who I am. I'm doing it right now, and I like that. And I like who I am. That's all the more reason to be good to myself.

On this journey, I wanted to understand myself better. I learned that I'm more than what I've been told, and more than what I thought of myself. I discovered how amazing I really can be when I put myself in the right situations, surround myself with the right people, and step up to challenges.

When I went to my first roller derby practice, I got hurt because I didn't fall properly. What a great metaphor for my life experience – I can get up every time I fall, but oh boy do I resist the fall! The first skills we learn in roller derby are how to fall, and how to stop. Falls had been my bane for a while. Once I practiced falling (lots of times) properly, it became more natural. I could always get up, and I just needed to work on falling, over and over again, until my muscle memory kicked in and it became a solid skill. It still sucks to fall, but I've learned to let my body go with it, instead of have an "oh shit!" moment and resist it. Those "oh shit!" moments, for me, have caused injuries (some foreshadowing here!).

In life, I've fallen many times. I stayed down; staying down was familiar. But what staying down meant for me is that I allowed the downward spiral, I kept making unhealthy choices, gaining weight, and ultimately let myself get sick. Once I had enough, it was time to change—it was time to get back up. I knew I could; I know that about myself. I just had to allow myself to DO it!

So again, when I'm asked "can you believe who that was?" or told "that's not even you anymore!" I still reply "You're damn right that is me! THAT is the woman who lost all the excess fat!!!"

Once more, it's not about what I did, it's about why, and how I did it!

Questions:
List three accomplishments you're proud of:
1)
2)
3)
What is something you'd like to discover about yourself?

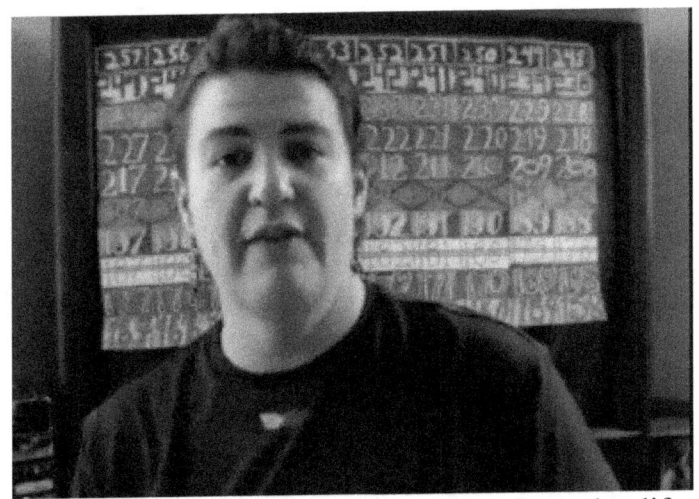

Reason #12 – <u>Learning moderation transcends into other life aspects</u>
Recorded on December 5, 2012

How we do one thing is how we do everything.

When we start eating healthier and tracking our nutrition, that accountability is a habit that touches various facets of our lives. We find consistent results with consistent healthy habits in mind, body and spirit. This helps mitigate stress.

When we're excessively stressed, it triggers excessive habits. When we find inner peace and calm, we're smart about decisions we make, and are less likely to fall into self-destructive patterns, such as pigging out on a gallon of ice cream while phoning an abusive ex.

We cannot change what comes our way, but we can change how we respond.

When we track our nutrition, it's amazing how that affects our ability to create and stick with a financial budget. When we work out more, we're less likely to go overboard on our meals and how we eat. When we allow ourselves to love and accept ourselves, people love and accept us as well.

It may never be perfect, but it's good, and that is worth the effort!

Activity:

Get together with some friends or family and schedule a salad party (stick with me, this will be totally fun, creative, and tasty)! Arrange a list of suggested items and have everyone sign up to bring something. Be sure to include the following on your list: greens, vegetables, proteins (meats and vegetarian options), dressings, mix-ins, and healthy sides. You'll be amazed how fun and interesting this is! Schedule these types of get-togethers monthly, and as you get really good at it, create a theme. For instance, a healthy taco salad themed party: the sign-up sheet includes lean taco meat, shredded lettuces, pico de gallo, cilantro, lime, jalapenos, olives, shredded cheese (go easy on the cheese, stick to the serving sizes), beans, and a fruit salad for dessert. When everyone arrives with their contributions, set the food on a table with plates and silverware, and everyone gets to make their own plates!

It's a sneaky way of having a healthy pot luck, and you get to control the ingredients by creating a sign-up list with only healthy ingredients. Make it a point to remind your guests that you're eating healthy and want them to join you in this meal for fun, support, and to share in a great experience together!

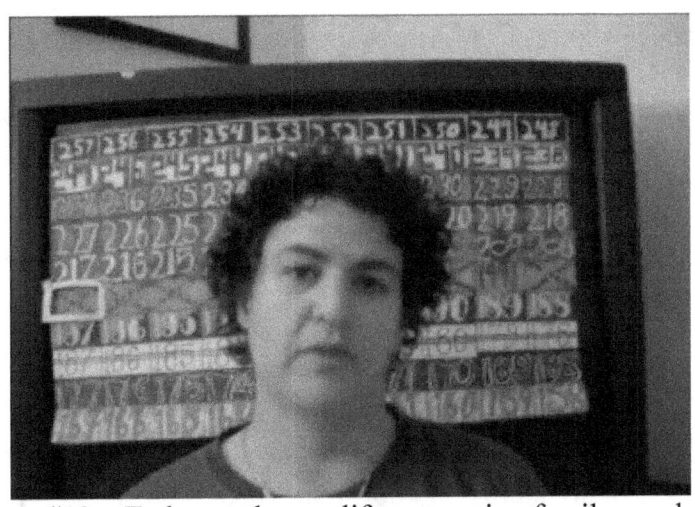

Reason #13 – <u>To have a longer lifespan, enjoy family, goals, etc.</u>
Recorded on December 6, 2012
Weight: 207 pounds

When I finally started dating (I'd repressed my sexuality for nearly 30 years, so it took me a while to get out there…plus I was hiding under 100 pounds of excess fat), I realized that I do ultimately want to get married and have a family.

Through my experience, I've witnessed that the best way to attract the best things into our lives is by treating ourselves how we want to be treated. In previous relationships, I did too much, with little or no reciprocity. Getting out of a relationship was a HUGE catalyst for my lifestyle transition – I finally came to understand that people will only treat us as well as we treat ourselves, and as well as we ALLOW them to. I was not allowing myself to be treated well before, because I wasn't treating myself well.

I had an ongoing pattern of bad decision-making when it came to selecting dating partners, so I wanted to take a step away to focus on healing myself so I wouldn't openly expose myself to more abuse from others and from myself. I wanted to do better. I wanted to *BE* better.

It was a huge step for me to finally say that that I want to get married, and that I deserve it. Even now, I struggle with accepting that there's some great stuff here, and that when the time is right, whoever she is, she'll find her way into my life and into my heart. That may be a year from now, many years from now, and maybe that person is just myself. However it happens, I know that first and foremost, I want to be healthy, happy and inwardly fulfilled before attracting, and finally bringing, that special someone into my life.

Since I want the happy ending and a long, healthy, and prosperous life with a wife, I want to take care of myself so that I can fully enjoy it. I want to share the rewards of my success with my wife and our family. As I progress in my journey, I know that whoever she is, she is out there, doing the same for herself. While she's doing her work, I'm doing mine. I'm worth it, and totally worth the wait. So is she!

Assignment:
Write a letter to your family, expressing your love, gratitude and appreciation for them. Sincerely tell them how they've impacted your life, and how you want to be the best version of yourself to be an example for them. Remind them that they are a gift, and every day you feel (happy, grateful, blessed, etc.) to have them in your lift. Tell them what your dreams are for the future, and what roles they play in your dream.

You have the option to read this letter to them, or to use this master letter as a reference when writing individual letters to each family member you'd like to write to. Then, either read their letter to them, or surprise each of them with a hand-written card or note. Put it in their lunches, a jacket or pants pocket, or in their rooms.

So often we spend our time complaining and telling our families the bad stuff. Take a moment and write for the sake of telling them you love them, and that you want to be around for a long time to keep loving them!

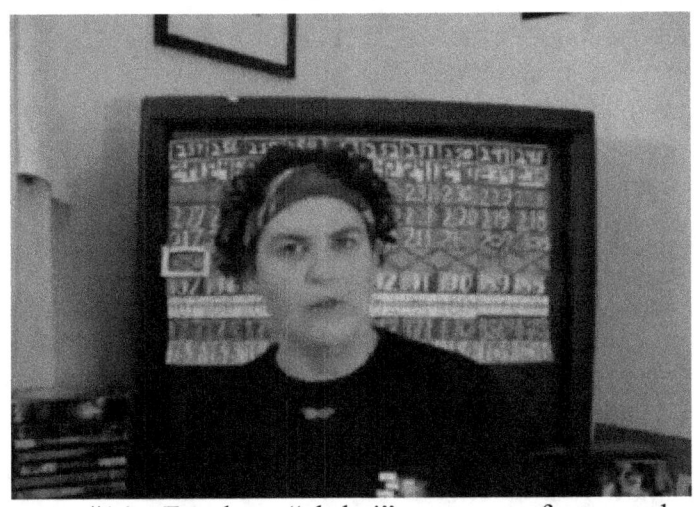

Reason #14 – <u>For those "ah-ha!" moments after a workout</u>
Recorded on December 6, 2012
Weight: 207 pounds

From the video for this reason:
We fear something more than the actual outcome…just do the best that you can, and keep going.

Whenever we work hard at something particularly challenging, it will make us grow in some way, shape or form. Even when we falter, something will be gained from the experience. We fall, we piss, we moan, and then we get back up and give it another shot.

It will ALWAYS be hard, but it will ALWAYS be worth it. When we invest in ourselves and put the work in, the relief is euphoric. The feeling is indescribable.

So many great, yet short-lived moments happen after completing a challenge: Savasana after a yoga practice, runner's high, an orgasm after sex, or that one cheat meal or cheat day per week that we allow ourselves. These moments are meant to be savored, because we've worked so hard for them, and especially because we earned them. It's a high that cannot be purchased, it cannot be taken; it can only be earned.

Working out may not pay the bills, get all the work done, or completely silence the voices in our heads that say mean things to us, but for a few moments, it makes the little things matter the most and the troubling things matter the least.

Challenge:
Read this reason again while doing jumping jacks!
After you re-read the reason and do the jacks, do five push-ups! You may keep your knees down if it is painful to do the five push-ups without assistance. Once you've hit five, see how many more you can do!
Make some notes in your journal, describing how it felt to do these things, and how you felt after.

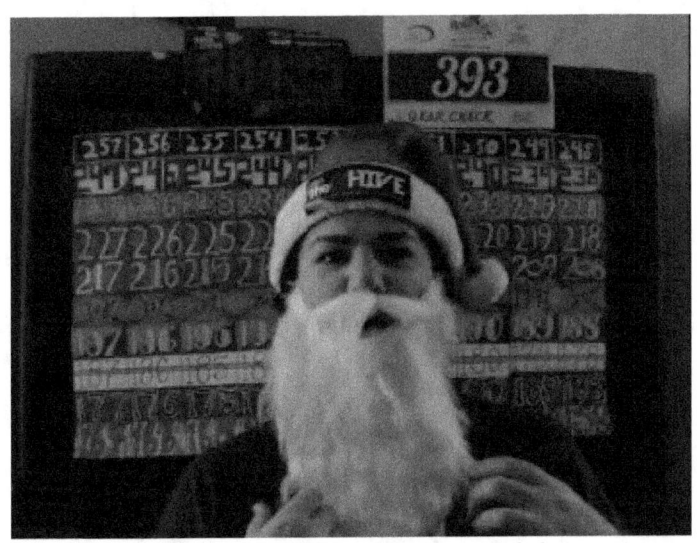

Reason #15 – <u>To blow off steam and de-stress</u>
Recorded on December 10, 2012
Weight: 213 pounds

Exercise generates endorphins, and endorphins make us happy! I have experienced this with *every* workout. This natural high is amazing, and though it can be difficult getting psyched up and dressed for a workout, the reward is always better than the excuses.

The hardest part about getting into a fitness routine is getting started, whether it's the first workout ever, or the workout of the day.

Working out and eating healthier helped me realize how instrumental healthy habits are in my healing, and I was experiencing the results in my body, my mind, and my spirit. Working out has lifted my spirits every day. It makes me feel better about myself and about my life, thanks to the magic of an endorphin rush from a workout, the sense of pride and accomplishment that comes from eating healthy, and the relief that comes from living a healthy lifestyle as opposed to the life I was living before.

In the past, I'd eat a pint (sometimes two) of ice cream when I was feeling sad. This felt good in the moment, but ultimately it would always lead to regret (and tighter clothes), leading to even more stress. Now I get to work off stress in yoga, or by roller skating, or by teaching a fitness class. After these activities, I get to take a hot shower or a bubble bath. There's no regret there! The best part? ALL of these activities are stress-busters! I will always be recovering from a lifetime of obesity. This is a lesson I keep in mind every single day. Watching the video for this reason and writing this out is yet another reminder to stick with it, keep going, and that it may be hard, but the results are always worth it.

Assignment:
You'll need a dry-erase board, poster board, big calendar sheet (or seven sheets of paper put together), and your notebook. In your notebook, write down a goal you'd like to achieve for the week. One simple, clear, and attainable goal. Some examples are: work out for 3 days, make lunches every day for the week, drink 8 glasses of water per day, get 8 hours rest every night, and so on.

Once you've chosen your goal, plan that one thing into your week. Be sure to include your wake-up times, your meals, when you work, your responsibilities and obligations, and your recreational, social, and family time. It's best to be consistent with what time you plan your goal activity each day.

When you've completed your calendar, put it in a place you'll see it every day, and/or a place you'll see it as soon as you get out of bed. Look at it daily, and throughout the day. Take a picture of it with your phone and look at the picture regularly.

After you've had a successful week achieving this goal (which may require several attempts), go for three more weeks, following this weekly plan. Once you've been successful at this for a month, add on another goal in the same style next month! Remember, I said add on – you're going to keep up this habit and build a new one as well!

This is a great way to integrate habits gradually for sustainable results!

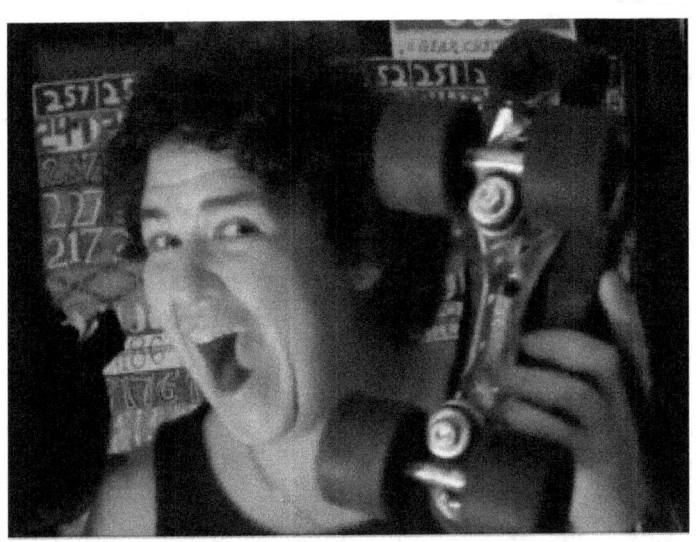

Reason #16 – <u>To keep my menstrual cycle normal</u>
Recorded on December 5, 2012
Weight: 211 pounds

From the video for this reason:
What I really appreciate about this journey is feeling it here and here...and making the connection that I'm allowed to have this...it's going to happen...I don't know where we're going, but it's going to be amazing.

It had taken some time before I had finally gotten to embrace the beauty in the journey, instead of being wholly fixated on the end result. Truly, I kept thinking about having a "perfect" body. Thankfully, my focus has shifted to loving the journey. Even now, after hitting my goal, I still think about that perfect body, but in all truth, my body is exactly what it needs to be. Even if there's loose skin, scars, stretch marks and "flaws", it serves me. My body does exactly what it needs to do, thanks to conditioning. What's most important, truly, is what's going on inside.

Not just pertaining to my ovaries and female parts, but what's going on in my mind, and in my spiritual connections.

This journey is all about finding self-love. I've grown to accept who I am and allow myself to be my full, authentic self. That meant shedding the thoughts, ideas, and habits that were limiting me. Those thoughts stressed me out. It was stress that jacked up my menstrual cycle.

There has only been one instance since hitting my goal that my period's timing was off, and it was when I was going through an unbearable and stressful work situation, specifically the environment.

That's a whole different Smashing Success Story! Just like my healthy lifestyle transition, it also has a happy ending!

Getting healthy did, indeed, fix my menstrual cycle. It also helped me move on from that horrifying work situation.

There's a silver lining and happy ending to it all!

Speaking of happy things, in the video for this reason, I'm super excited because I finally got a pair of roller skates, and I finished the artwork on my helmet!

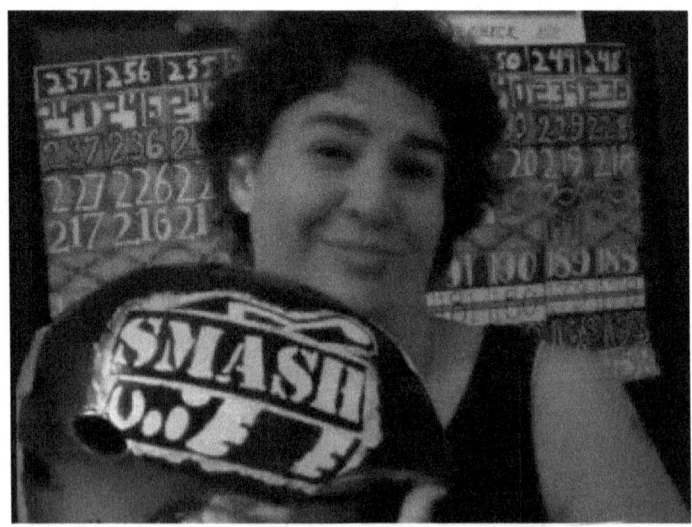

SMASH TANK IN THE HOUSE!!!

The little things really do add up! My motivation was through the roof!

Questions:
What are your major sources of stress?
How do you manage your stress?
How would you benefit from reducing the stress in your life?
Has your health been affected by the stress in your life? How so?

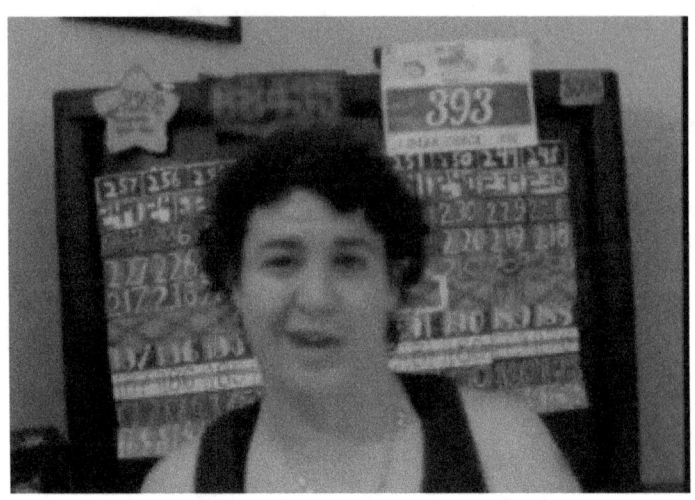

Reason #17 – <u>So I can get more body art</u>
Recorded on January 10, 2013
Weight: 201 pounds

This is great reminder that the difficult things are always worth it, just like getting a tattoo. Tattoos hurt. They're annoying, and we have to earn our tattoos, just like we earn the stories they tell.

The difficult things, of course, yield the greatest rewards! Tattoos are a lot like breeding rabbits – it doesn't stop with just one, and oh boy how they add up! As soon as I got my pin-up girl reward tattoo, I had seven more tattoos planned.

SEVEN.

Again, it's because the beauty is in the journey, not the destination. We remember stories from experiences, not just the end result. Ideally, getting tattooed is a wonderful experience; tattoo artists have amazing stories and it's great to talk through it. I've had the amazing good fortune of having talented tattoo artists who are also excellent conversationalists!

Here's the pin-up girl tattoo I got when I lost 50 pounds and hit my half-way mark!

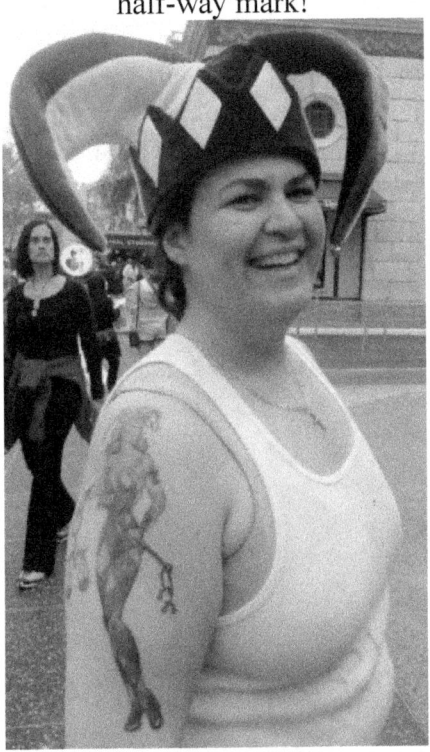

I've since gotten two more tattoos since then…

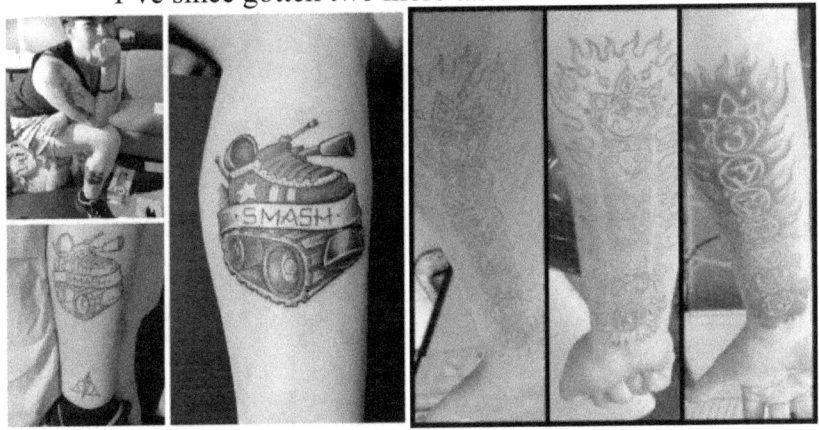

…six more to go!

Assignment:

Find at least three things on your body that tell a story, and think about how you got them. Scars are especially interesting! Consider the circumstances that brought about that feature (it can be the color of your eyes, who you inherited that from, the color of your hair, a surgical scar, freckles and so on). Write about at least three of these features, and feel free to write as much as you'd like about them, and for as many features as you can think of. Spend at least 20 minutes on this assignment.

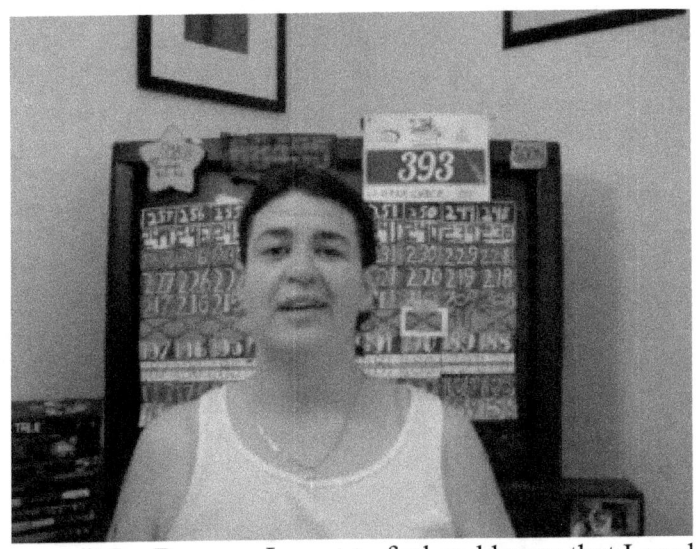

Reason #18 – <u>Because I want to feel and know that I am hot</u>
Recorded on January 14, 2013
Weight: 200 pounds

People are drawn to confident people; we all want to feel confident and when we come across someone who seems confident, we are naturally attracted to them.

There's something magical about the confidence that comes from earning something by working hard for it. Sure, when we're looking and feeling fit it's conveyed in our body language and attitude, but it's more about how it makes us *feel,* and that great feeling is very appealing. People pick up on it, and confidence itself is naturally attractive.

Looking great is a fantastic dividend of making the lifestyle transition. However, it's really about the changes it causes within. Knowing that I earned this has been a huge reward that keeps me going. Now, I feel good because I treat myself well. I look good for me; I'm the one looking in the mirror now and I feel the validation.

When I take care of myself, I feel good. Over the course of my life, I sure did put my body and heart through a lot of abuse, some of it as a way to protect myself from others abusing me (I thought if I was big, no one would be attracted to me and wouldn't be able to hurt me – and I was dead wrong about that), and some of it was to punish myself.

I had to change my thoughts, and by changing my thoughts, I changed my life.

When we do it for the sake of impressing others, we become dependent on their input and that validation. Validation only lasts so long when it's external; it's eternal when it comes internally!

Questions:
What makes you feel sexy?
What are you attracted to?
How do you see yourself benefiting from feeling hot and attractive?
What are some of your features that you like?

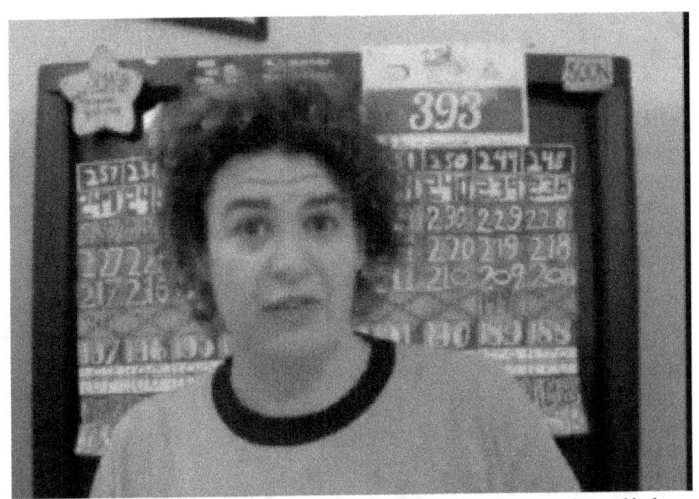

Reason #19 – <u>So I can dress super cute and stylish</u>
Recorded on May 15, 2013
Weight: 182

When I wrote my list, I legitimately thought that being fitter would make me want to dress cuter. I wore a few dresses from time to time, and I never felt comfortable in them.

I really thought I'd want to dress in feminine attire; I was treated better when I would wear dresses as opposed to wearing slacks and a polo shirt. The day after I wore a dress I was asked, "Why aren't you dressed cute today?"

Can't I just be cute without the dress?! Come on!

This was another reason I wrote while I was still seeking external validation. Again, the reasons were written when I was much heavier, and these were the ideas I had about what it would look and feel like once I had a fit physique.

A lot had happened in the gap of time between recording the videos for Reason #18 and Reason #19. I had broken my ankle, and I was so, so upset about how it would affect my workouts. It was also having a HUGE impact on my work life. People were saying derogatory things to me. My work duties had been modified. It was the second time I was experiencing discrimination, even after I addressed the issue with my boss at the time. I was angry quite often, partially because of the injury and how it limited me, and especially about how I was being treated. Things were NOT going my way at that time.

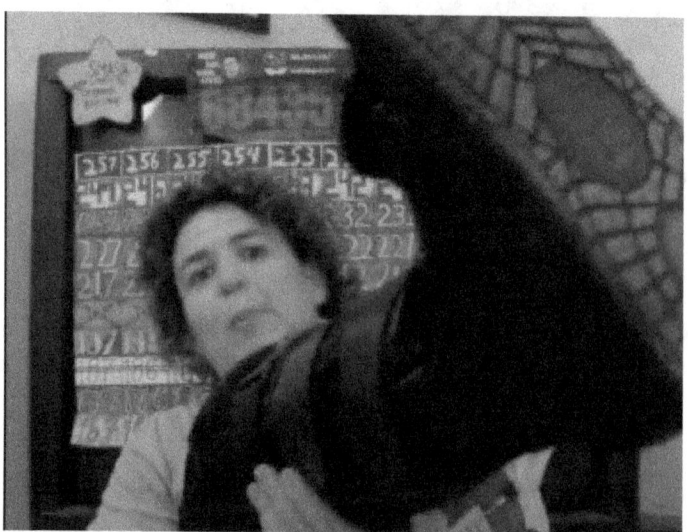
Not the kind of stylish boot I had in mind…

However, I was sticking with healthy eating and working out. I limited my workouts to solely upper-body strengthening, and I was in the gym at least four days per week, lifting weights and fine-tuning my strength training regimen.

So, for a little bit, I felt bad for myself, and I let it get to me. I was angry, and I definitely had a bad attitude. I did the last thing I wanted to do – I let that bullshit get to me, and I reacted in anger. I would vent by cursing at people behind closed doors, or when I'd put them on hold during a phone call. Those reactions were not how I wanted to feel nor, how I wanted to behave.

After a while though, I finally realized that there are still PLENTY of things I could do, and I focused my efforts and attention there, instead of on what I could not do. For instance, though I couldn't drive yet, I was able to spend more time with friends by asking for and receiving help with transportation (asking for help...wow that was a tough one. So, this experience also helped me develop that skill!). I couldn't run on a treadmill, so I put a lot of focus on developing more upper body strength. It actually presented an amazing opportunity to revolutionize my strength training routine!

This injury was by far one of the best learning experiences I've had. It helped me develop more compassion for people with challenges, especially life-long challenges. My experience was temporary, but I realized that is not the case for many people. What was a challenge for me for several months could be someone's LIFE experience.

We all have a choice – to fall into the darkness and let it consume us, or to find the light within and to rise from the darkness. Do I want to be a victim, or a victor?

I choose victory.

This injury was a humbling learning experience for me, and though I still have some post-traumatic feelings that linger, just like the scars and the hardware that's now a permanent part of my body (come on, bionic parts are damn sexy), I am grateful for what I learned in the experience.

Now, I get to use this experience to encourage and uplift others.

It may seem so little, something as simple as a broken ankle. However, that broken ankle shifted my perspective. It really changed my life, and it galvanized me as a person, an athlete, a professional, and as a skater.

To this day I'm still affected by this injury. It's a part of my story, a part of my life, and will be a part of my legacy.

But with a name like Smash Tank, there isn't much that can keep me down for long!

Assignment:
Find an outfit you like in the next size down. It can be new, on clearance, or found at a thrift store. Write a note with the date a month from the day you purchased it, and stick the note on the outfit. On that day, try it on! Take pictures and journal the experience!

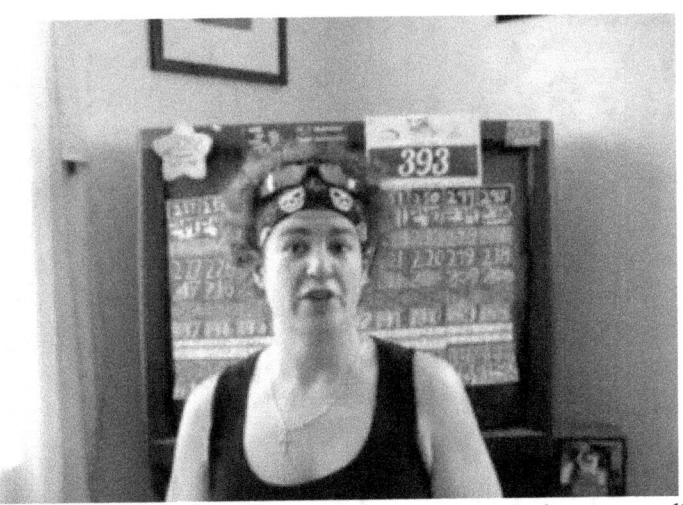

Reason #20 – <u>So my clothes fit right and I don't have to pull and stretch on them</u>
Recorded on May 18, 2013

Getting fit and shredding body fat made me feel more comfortable in my clothes, and I started wearing clothes that were fitted and much more flattering. Wearing properly fitted clothes means that now I don't need to tug at them. Every now and then I'll still catch myself pulling at my clothes, and it's just an unconscious tick, left over from a lifetime of pulling and stretching my clothes.

Good habits in nutrition and fitness have made it easier to stay within a size range...for the most part. Hey, I'm a woman, and we do fluctuate in size from time to time, especially during certain times of each month. I know myself well enough to hang onto things a size up when I stray from my plan from time to time. It happens. This way, I don't have to worry about wearing things that don't fit me right, and I don't have to keep buying different clothes every time I have a shift.

It's awesome to sit down and not worry about my clothes tugging at me. My old issue used to be when they would tug at my belly, and now, if anything, they can be tight across my shoulders, back and chest due to my muscle mass (I intended to build muscle, and oh boy did I!).

Activity:

Go to your closet and dresser, and take out anything that you haven't worn in the past 12 months. Even if there is an outfit you're hanging onto, get rid of it. You deserve a new one when you've hit your milestones. Donate these clothes to charity. For the remainder of the things in your closet, switch the direction of the hangers. When you wear something and have washed and dried it, put it back on the hanger and put the hanger in the original direction. At the end of six months, get rid of the clothes that are on hangers in the opposite direction! Do this every 6 months, getting rid of old clothes, things you no longer wear, and things that are at least two sizes too big!

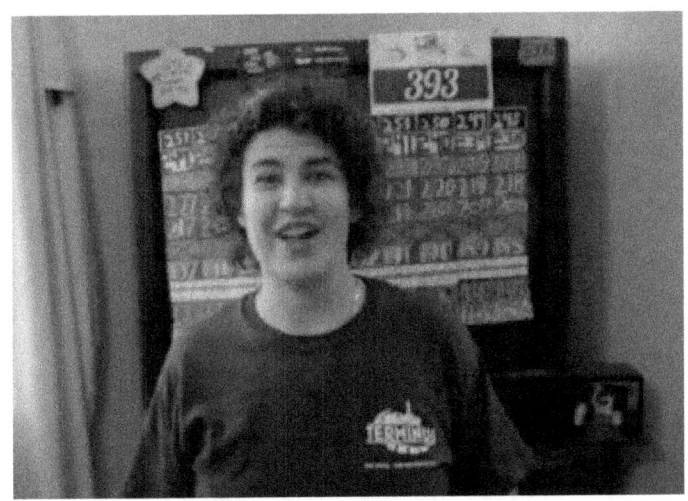
Reason #21 – <u>Shock value!</u>
Recorded on May 21, 2013

I LOVE showing people my "before" pictures, and I love running into folks that haven't seen me in a long time. Their reactions are priceless! It is amazing to see how happy people are when we succeed at something! I've come to witness that it inspires them and gives them hope to carry on with their own journeys and pursue their own goals.

When we set goals, we come up with an action plan, and actions create habits. Habits create results. It's a simple formula. There are few things as powerful and motivational as results.

Though the formula is simple, the trick is creating the habits. As I'm writing this, I'm also drafting action plans to help folks create habits to reach their next level of potential. This comes from experience, and with experience comes mistakes, lessons learned, and the next round of action steps to continue building great habits!

From the video for this reason:
This whole journey is a learning process, of course it's interesting. A lot of new things pop up.

For so long I was my own worst enemy, taking it out on myself when something happened, and incessantly blaming myself when I'd make a mistake, or when people said hurtful things to me. Now, I know better. I still struggle with it sometimes, but my habits have changed, and that alone is shocking to me.

It's great to pleasantly surprise people, and it's pretty awesome when we can surprise ourselves!

Questions:
In what ways have you surprised yourself?
How have you surprised others?
What have you accomplished that you were afraid, doubtful, or skeptical about?

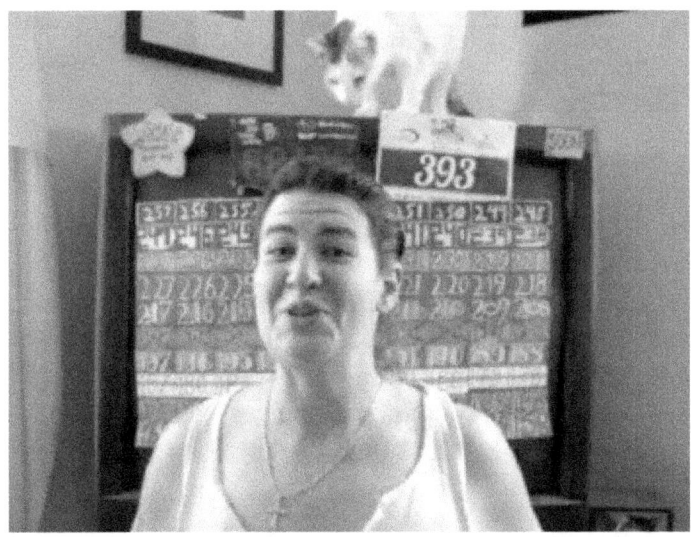

Reason #22 – <u>To be even more proud of myself</u>
Recorded on May 22, 2013

This is a day-to-day process, and I am proud of all I have done. I'm proud of myself every time I complete a workout, when I plan my meals, and when I stick to my plan for the day (especially my meal plans). However, I'm no angel, and I'm certainly not perfect. Mistakes have been some of the best lessons, and even when we're good at something, we can still fall back on old habits. That word right there is the key – habits.

Excellence is a habit. Happiness is a habit. Eating well is a habit.

Taking care of ourselves is a habit.

Loving ourselves is a habit.

There's this contrasting duality, a dichotomy that I experience, that I've observed in many others as well. I'm both insecure about myself, and proud of the things I've done. One comes from emotion, the other comes from logic. There's also the ego. It feeds incessantly, craves all, and is never satisfied. Then, there's the heart. It is grateful for everything, both the good and what appears to be bad.

There are moments when I'm just grateful for what I've accomplished, proud of what my body is capable of, and happy that I generally make good nutritional decisions.

Assignment:
Write one of your favorite stories that you tell people. It can be something you're proud of, like how well-behaved your kids are, how you learned to cook your favorite meal, the courage it took to ask your boss for a raise, how you secured your dream job, or whatever else you think of. Spend at least 20 minutes writing about this experience, what you did, and why you're proud of yourself for achieving this.

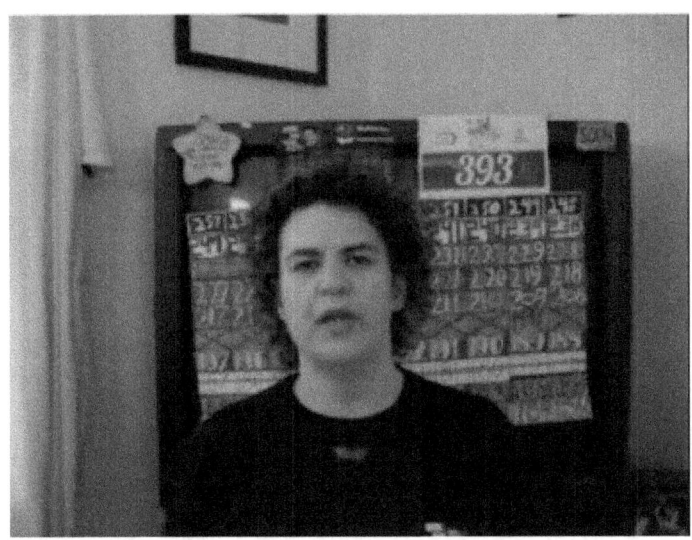

Reason #23 – <u>Because I DESERVE it!</u>
Recorded on May 23, 2013

Our purpose in life is more than just mere survival – we are destined to grow, prosper, and share what we have to spread it around. Wealth begets wealth. Greed begets greed – the more people steal and hoard, the more they continue to do it. We come to deserve great things by working for it (instead of stealing it) and sharing it (instead of hoarding it) with those who appreciate it.

Simple to visualize, yes. Easy to do, perhaps no. However, it's worth it. It can be done when we stick to simple things. When we listen to our hearts, we transition from how things *should* be to how they *are*. When we listen to our egos, it just gets in the way. When we accept things as they are, we accept ourselves. Then, we can truly see that we deserve only good things.

Anger, addiction, obesity, whatever it is we're struggling with, we take steps, each day, one day at a time.

So, easy does it, kiddo. You deserve greatness!

From the video for this reason:

There are things in this life that I deserve. I deserve a good life, I deserve to be comfortable, I deserve to feel peaceful, I deserve love, I deserve a good home, I deserve a great job, I deserve great means to get around, I deserve a healthy body, I deserve a healthy life, I deserve to take care of myself. Those are the things in my immediate circle of responsibility...those are the things that I am in control of, and if I'm not happy with it, I can change it.

Activity:

Get a stack of index cards, colored markers, pens, crayons or whatever you like to draw and write with. Feel free to get stickers and other embellishments! On each card, write a phrase and decorate your card. Write empowering, happy phrases, and create beautiful, colorful and bright cards. Place one card in each of the following: your mirror(s), your refrigerator, your pantry, your cupboard, the dashboard of your car, your work space, your lounging area (coffee table, by the couch and/or television, etc.), by your bed (lamp or nightstand), your closet and your dresser. Let the phrase be appropriate for the location – fulfilled on the card on the refrigerator, beautiful on the mirror card(s), safe/mindful/aware for the dashboard, grateful on the card by your bed and so forth. Let these cards serve as positive triggers, and when you see them, meditate on why you deserve to feel these things. Take your time on each card, and on finding the right phrase for each!

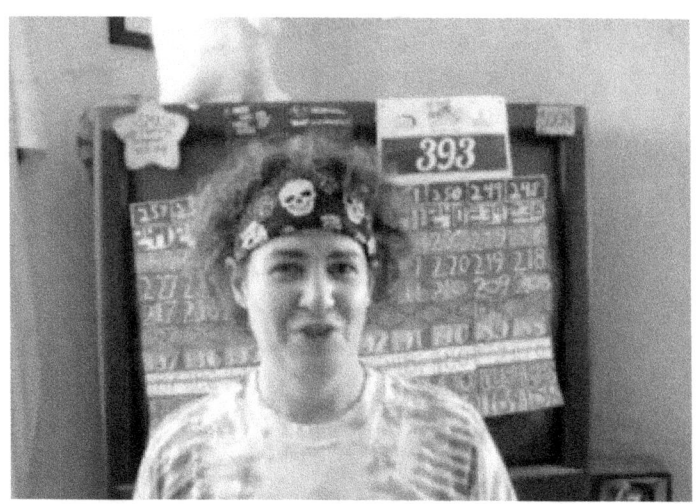

Reason #24 – <u>Because I WANT to!</u>
Recorded on May 25, 2013

I only want the best for myself and for our world. That is my heart's desire – to uplift people, to share for the sake of empowerment, and to raise people up. We all know how much it sucks to be put down.

I WANT to live a healthy life, for myself and for you!

My story comes from the heart, and when I listen to my heart and to other people, I find commonalities with EVERYONE I meet. I want to write, speak, and share my story and empower people to smash their goals as well. I could not have done this alone, and I want people to know they're not alone.

The "want" I talk about in this reason is a feeling based in desire. Desire can be both a good thing and a bad thing. <u>Eckhart Tolle</u> writes on his blog that "*It's been said there are two ways of being unhappy: One is not getting what you want, and the other is getting what you want.*"

So, why pursue a desire?

It depends on where it comes from. Is it an ego-based desire ("I want to do this so people will like my body and want me") or does it come from the heart ("I want to do this to build community, lift people up and inspire them to reach their goals")?

This is all about sharing and creating community, to build people up instead of tearing them down (confidence versus competition). To be a fully integrated person, we must be willing to step up and be champions, and then share the torch with others. When we can stand proudly and claim "I DID IT!" it should be for the sake of lighting as many candles as we can, not steal thunder from people around us.

May we all find authentic warriors who want the best for everyone, and who strive to become their best selves instead of compete with others.

Assignment:
Take five deep, mindful and cleansing breaths, inhaling to full capacity through your nose. Take long, slow, deep exhales through your nose, slower than the inhale. After your five cycles of breath, grab your notebook and write a list of 20 things you want to happen in your life, as fast as you can. Once you've hit 20, on the back of that sheet of paper or on the next page, write down a list of 20 things you want gone from your life. These can be anything that comes to mind. It can be as simple as "to spend more time in prayer" or something silly like "a big fat stack of bananas"! Just let it flow. You should feel uplifted and inspired after completing this assignment. If there are any resentments or bad feelings, come back to your breathing and keep going. It doesn't have to be perfect, and it should feel cleansing, empowering and cathartic.

After you've completed both lists, do five more cycles of breath, meditating on your heart's desires and being grateful for the work and this time you're taking to invest in yourself.

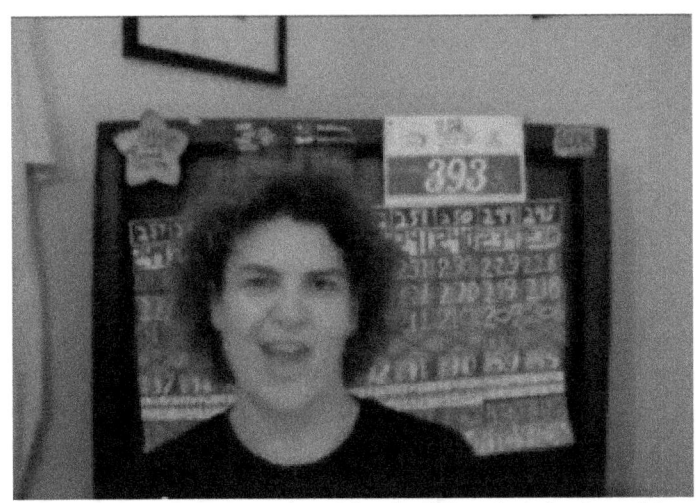

Reason #25 – <u>Because under this shell is a hot body with small shoulders, a smokin' ass, and great legs</u>
Recorded in May 2013

I really have no clue what led me to believe that I had a hot body under the excess fat I was carrying around—Perhaps memories of middle school, when I was riding my bicycle regularly, active in sports, and involved in martial arts. There was a brief stint in my adolescence where I was lifting weights for a bit and was eating in moderation. As a child, I went from being a picky eater to eating all of my emotions, then I was an active adolescent, and then around 16 years old, I took a drastic turn toward obesity. That last part went on for about 20 years.

When I wrote this list, I had a goal in mind, and the impetus to go for it. When embarking on this, I had an image of an ideal body, and yet, when I hit my goal, I thought I still had to lose more weight. I thought I still had fat to trim off. In all truth, there may have been some fat to cut, but it's really the excess skin that's what flaps now (sometimes it claps!). I have little control over that. I've come to accept it. The way I see it, my body is giving me applause when I work out (I cracked myself up when I had this thought)!

Which goes to show it's not about how it looks, it's about the journey, the habits, the choices made, and how it feels. I used to think I'd feel validated by how people would treat me once I was "good-looking." I found I was actually a bit repulsed by the difference in how I was being treated. People seemed to like me more as a fit person, I was getting hit on, and I felt SO uncomfortable. People remarked on my looks, and it made me feel devalued as a person.

It's what's on the inside that matters. Even now when I consider dating someone, I want to get to know someone from the inside, not go for what I see on the outside.

I've learned that attraction goes WAY beyond looks.

I'm a woman of value, and yes, I do have some great physical attributes, and I will wholly admit that when I did FINALLY share myself with another person, I felt like a real super stud when she told me she loved my body. I gave a huge sigh of contentment and said, "Thank you. Thank you so much for appreciating this." It's great to have an awesome body, and it's super when that is appreciated. Though that's not the end-all, it's a great dividend. It's an even bigger bonus when we find someone that can appreciate all that there is on the inside as well as the outside.

But first, we must address what's on the inside, because that will help us accept ourselves as we are, not how we "should" be.

I will gladly admit though, my shoulders are toned and sculpted, my legs are pretty spectacular, and my ass is stellar! I've worked hard for this and I will continue to take care of myself, for life. I'm worth it. My body is worth it. I look and feel healthy!

Questions:
What are three physical features you like about yourself?
What are three things that you appreciate about yourself right now?

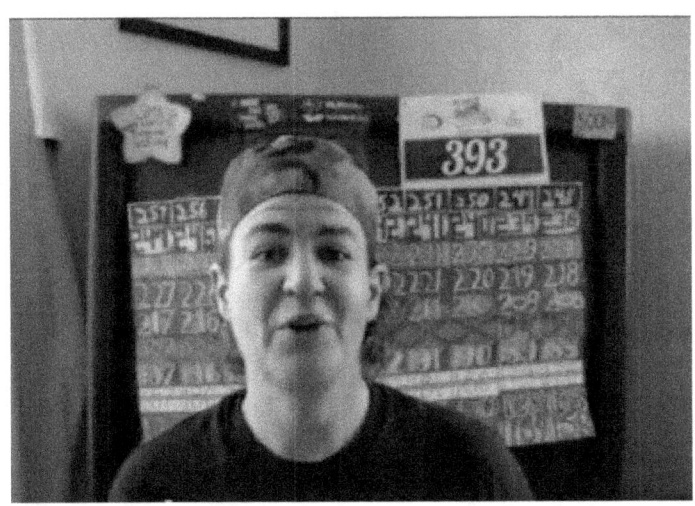
Reason #26 – <u>I know I can, that's why!</u>
Recorded on May 26, 2013

Writing these reasons was a huge step for me when this started. It seemed audacious to aspire to something so big, to think I could be a healthy and fit person after living a lifetime of hiding under a shell of excess fat. However, I believed then just as I believe now – when we aspire to something and listen to our hearts, we're already claiming it and just need to do the work to make it happen.

I've wanted to do this for a very, very long time. I just needed the right push.

From the video for this reason:
This is something I've always felt for myself, and I've always seen the future as successful. There are times I struggle with it, going, 'maybe I'm delusional, maybe this is my destiny.' I'm going with the latter…Just because I haven't had it doesn't mean that it's not going to happen. I just gotta make it a reality.

The biggest and best accomplishments seem impossible. In his book <u>Think and Grow Rich,</u> Napoleon Hill writes that "desire *backed by faith* knows no such word as impossible."

If there's anything I know to be truth, it's this – all it takes is faith, dedication, vision, hard work, inspiration, and good habits to persist through any challenge. Some days are harder than others. Some weeks are a challenge. Sometimes, I skip a workout. I'll drive past my favorite fast food restaurants and imagine ordering some of my old favorites. Sometimes...I actually do. This experience means more than just creating healthy habits in nutrition and exercise; it also means being okay with making mistakes. It's been over two years since I've had ice cream, and sometimes I drive past Dairy Queen wondering if I could have one more. What would it be like if I went back to eating lots of sugar, ice cream, candy bars and such? What would it be like if I had just *one last one*?

Thoughts are just that – they're thoughts. We can exercise some control over this, and the biggest thing we have power over is our actions.

So often I hear, "it's too hard" or "that's work," and you know what? Boo-freaking-hoo. The greats NEVER had it easy. They did things that no one else before them had done. That's what makes them legendary. The most influential and inspirational people didn't have it easy – they faced incredibly difficult hardships and paved new ways of overcoming them.

Every single day there are people working miracles. Just as I've lost 100 pounds and maintained a healthy lifestyle, there's someone out there (MANY actually) raising a child on his or her own. That's unfathomable to me, and so remarkably amazing. There are countless people living with terminal illness, and not dying from a disease, but LIVING with it. Folks from all walks of life find sobriety after a lifetime of use. Abuse victims learn to love. People who have lost everything still have *faith*.

We are not the product of what has happened to us, we are made by these things and how we've *overcome* them.

Unlike many internal conflicts, obesity is not something I could hide. I could stay in the closet (that lasted about 30 years), I could hide alcoholism by drinking alone at the end of the day when no one was around, I could avoid needy tendencies by staying single and abstaining from sex altogether, but none of these fixed the underlying problem.

Challenges forge us into who we really are. Life invariably will throw uncertainties, challenges, and obstacles our way. Just because we suffer doesn't mean we have to hurt – we can take something from it and turn it into something amazing. We can turn it around and make it part of our story, and then spread that message and hope to others.

We're stronger than our excuses and there isn't anything more powerful than will and choice. Nothing "makes" us do something, no one "makes us feel" anything. We are free and independent people, responsible for our own lives. We're autonomous. The more we listen with our hearts instead of our screaming egos, the more we can see how choice and opportunity line up so serendipitously.

THAT is our purpose, THAT is our destiny – to live in order to fulfill a higher purpose, and only we know that purpose by listening to our hearts and taking action.

It happens in moments; moments of faith, of will, of habit, and especially action.

Those moments mean *everything.*

Impossible is an excuse used by doubters and people who give up too easily. It's the creative people that find a way— they become inventors and mavericks by persisting and believing.

It takes courage to believe in something that we can't see. Faith isn't a crutch, it's strength. Faith is knowing that it will work, not knowing *how* it will work, but know that it WILL work.

This all started as an idea. I wanted it so badly, and I took action. Then, I started believing. I have yet to experience disappointment when I've believed I can do something and I've put in hard work to see it through. Things may not turn out how I expected them to, but every single time I embark on something I believe in, I get it. It doesn't happen right away, it happens over time and after a LOT of mistakes.

It all started because I believed I could. Then, I did it.

So can you!

Activity:
Invite some friends over that inspire, encourage, and support you. Give them all a guest book for them to put in their homes, and write something inside each of their guest books. Be sure you have one for yourself as well! Encourage them to all write something in your book that they're proud of you for. Every time you have guests over, invite them to write in your book! You'd be amazed to see the kind, supportive and generous things people will share with you!

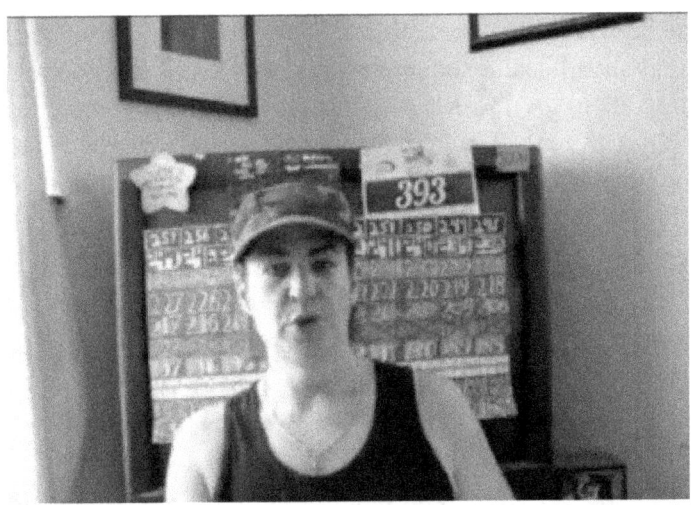

Reason #27 – <u>Because I want to be close to natural foods and this will do that</u>

Recorded on May 27, 2013

From early on— I'm talking the earliest I can recall— I've had a tumultuous relationship with food. I started dieting when I was about 8 years old. Meal replacement shake bullshit had been a part of my household for years. It was something that became such a struggle because, like many struggling with weight management and committing to a healthy lifestyle, the focus was on losing weight instead of healthy living.

Time and experience have taught me that food is always the winner. Fasts, meal replacements and other substitutes just didn't work in the long run. I'm grateful for the various diets and fasts that I've tried (like a raw food diet, the Paleolithic diets and juice fasts) because they got me to eat more natural, earth-based foods, but its whole food that has become a staple.

Sure, I'm STILL tempted by the constant barrage of quick, take-out, ready-made, amazing-smelling foods. Every time I drive home from teaching, I pass by a fried chicken restaurant that tests my will on a daily basis! I've worked hard, I'm sweaty and hungry, and that smell is SO tempting! There have been a couple times that I've caved, and each experience has taught me something. I know from experience that too much of that stuff has consequences, just as I know that too much restriction leads to total loss of self-control. Eating that stuff in very, *very* rare doses is okay. Going overboard just feels terrible. Maybe one day I can totally give it up.

When it comes to whole foods, there are rarely, if any, regrets. When we stock our shelves, refrigerators and pantries with healthy options, it saves us from impulsively eating too much of the wrong thing. When we arm ourselves with the right tools, we get the job done correctly!

Whole foods look amazing, taste great, and help our bodies operate optimally. There's a reason why whole food has been around since the age of civilization – it has always provided for us, will always be good for us, is bountiful, and fulfills us! Real food for the win!

Assignment:
Make a list of healthy, whole and natural foods that you like – fruits, vegetables, meats, snacks and such. Make another list of whole foods that you just do not like at all. Then, look up recipes that include the foods you've listed in your "like" list. Try at least three of these recipes that week, and buy the ingredients once you've gone over your list and researched the recipes. The best way to optimize your shopping is to look up recipes that have some of the same ingredients, and yet enough variety to keep things interesting!

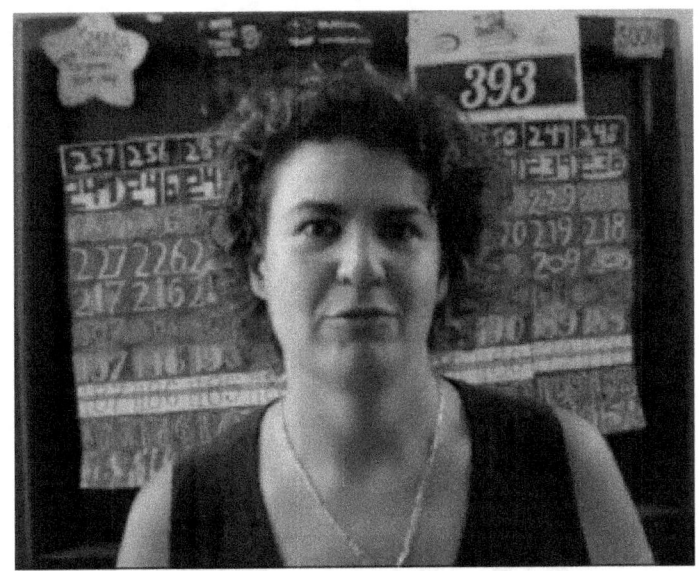

Reason #28 – <u>To manage my A.D.D.</u>
Recorded on May 28, 2013

A friend had shared with me how she took her son off of medication (he also has Attention Deficit Disorder) and treated him with clean, whole foods. His teachers and family noticed a HUGE difference. I have experienced this difference as well, and attribute it to eating clean and healthy foods, staying on top of my fitness, utilizing prayer and meditation, and staying present and focused on the moment.

Eating clean also helps me stay focused, and I know that's because I have less chemicals running through my system. Getting rid of sugary and processed foods helps my brain process things much more efficiently!

Having Attention Deficit Disorder is yet another facet of myself I struggled with for SO long. I now know this part of me will never go away, just like I can't outrun my past, I can't out-Christian my sexuality, and I can't out-smart my addiction. It is what it is, so I have learned to live with it.

Part of living with it is coming up with strategies to make my life more efficient. In addition to eating healthy and exercising regularly, I also found that it helps me stay present and focused when I sit in the "T" section (front and middle rows) of classes and meetings, avoid windows (OH PRETTY!), and silence my phone and put it out of sight and mind. Also, creating and sticking to daily action plans and to-dos lists have been instrumental.

Planning my day, having my meals prepared (or having prepared foods ready to go) keeps my distractions at bay, and I can then focus more on bigger tasks. A plan keeps me in line, and having healthy foods keeps my brain and body functioning fantastically!

Challenge:
Set a timer for one hour, and turn off music, television, computer and silence your phone. No books, no sleeping, no distractions and no talking at all. For this one hour, you are challenged to create space in your mind, your home and in your spirit for peace. If there is an area of your home that desperately needs organizing, this is the time to do it. Spend this time in prayer, meditation, taking a walk or a drive in a new area. Avoid anything that diverts your attention. Meditate on your goals and where you want to be. Spend this hour (and more if needed) on bettering your mind, your environment, and your spiritual connection. Focus, visualize, create space, and receive what you need in this time. Do this weekly!

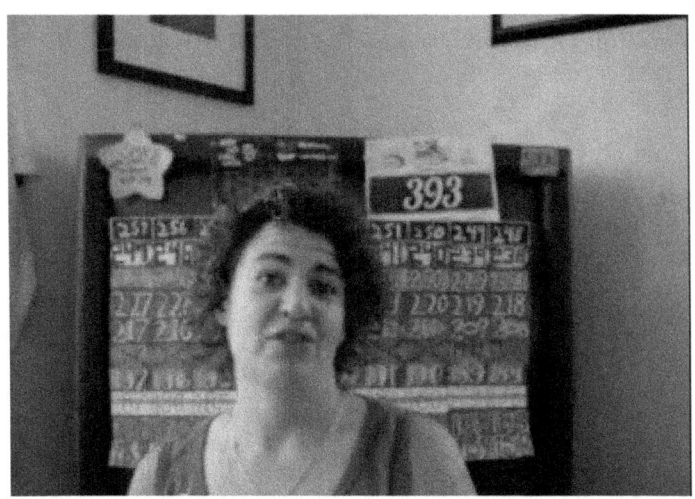

Reason #29 – <u>Because I want to develop better habits all around</u>
Recorded on May 29, 2013

Holding myself accountable is a big theme in my life, and of course, the phrase "how we do one thing is how we do everything" comes to mind again. So, with this reason, I knew that healthy habits in nutrition and exercise would lead to better habits altogether. How I consume calories is the same way I spend money – when I have a plan of action and a goal, I'm on point. When I have free reign, it's a mess! So, by finding a balance in my workouts and nutrition, I am prepared to be better in many areas of things in my life. Or better at, as we say, "adulting."

When I'm on a schedule, I do better about moderation and sticking to a regimen. When it's a workday (back when I had a regular job), that schedule helped me delegate specific times for specific things and to prepare meals to stay on track. On my days off work, I have a successful day when I plan my day in advance, just like I do for workdays. When my activities and meals are planned, I'm less likely to veer off track.

From the video for this reason:
Developing healthy habits is about doing it right now, not waiting until Monday, or New Year's, or before a wedding. It's a conscious choice

83

that happens right now…it's a matter of making gradual, sustainable changes for life.

Balance and moderation have truly touched many facets of my life, and this experience revolutionized my habits, attitudes and overall actions. What a great multipurpose tool kit!

Habits don't just miraculously, magically appear because we want them to. If we want something, we need to plan for it. Dreaming and wishing are good and well, but devising a plan and strategies is what helps bring our dreams and wishes into reality. If we don't take the necessary steps from desiring an outcome to actually planning how to work toward that outcome, then we're going to let ourselves down.

I wish I could give everyone a magical wish-granting fairy. I really wish I could. However, I don't have that power (yet). Instead, I want to empower you to be your own wish-granting fairy (or if you want something more masculine, imagine a genie). Turn your goal into action steps by breaking it down into monthly, weekly, and then daily tasks. That's how we take on a huge endeavor – one step at a time. Create a schedule and stick to it.

Assignment:
Are you sticking to your weekly plan from Reason #15? It doesn't have to be perfect, however, we should work our plan and plan our work. Come back to the planning phase, and plan your week. It doesn't have to start on a Monday – start now. Plan for these essential activities: meal preparation, eating, working, exercising, spiritual practices, and reviewing your goals, notes, and journal logs. Review and look for productivity gaps and any patterns that may compromise your goals. Come up with action plans to resolve these. Learn from each experience and take a few moments to practice gratitude for the time and energy you're putting into this!

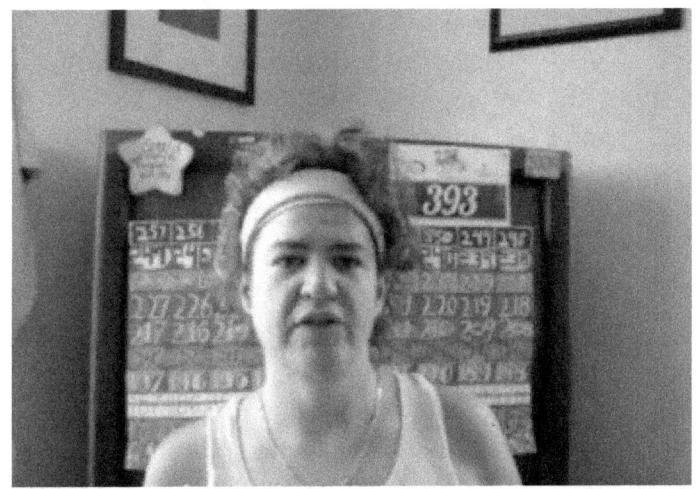

Reason #30 – <u>To find moments of peace in my workouts</u>
Recorded on June 2, 2013

The best part of hard work is when it's done! There are some amazing moments during the challenge, but the best feeling is the relief when it's over. It feels great to accomplish something! I love the endorphin rush of a great workout, and after all that labor and sweat, that glow and pride remind me that I did it, yet again. It's always hard to get started, and it's always worth it in the end!

Sense a theme here? I say versions of that quote repeatedly. Just like group fitness and yoga instructors give alignment and form cues, even if they're reiterations of cues they've already said, it's because we often forget the simple things (like keep your shoulders back, remember to breathe, bend your knees). We need to be reminded. If you're reading this book, maybe you're like me. Maybe hearing something over and over didn't quite sink in the other times, but there's that *one time* that it really touched you. As the saying goes, "when the student is ready, the master will appear" (that's from various paraphrased quotes credited to Buddha).

Working out is a reward in and of itself, and the feelings it creates are an amazing high. I can't sell you on workouts, and I can't promise it'll make you feel a certain way, just as I can't tell you how a specific drug will make you feel. I can tell you how it makes ME feel, and working out makes me feel like a rock star! After I finish a great lifting session, my muscles feel and look more defined, and that makes me feel like I'm (quite frankly) hot. I feel good, and I feel like I look good! After I finish an endurance workout (like cycling or roller skating), the endorphin rush is a combination of peace-inducing, energizing, and a feeling of HUGE relief.

It's hard work to exercise, and at the end, I feel proud that I've done it, and I know that I can do it again. It's a confidence-builder. It creates lasting results. It inspires me to keep going. Plus one of my absolute favorite things in life is a hot, steamy shower. After a great workout, I totally revel in that hot shower! That is an amazing reward just by itself!

We all have that option, and it's not about doing crazy intensive stuff all the time. It's about finding several things you enjoy, and trying new things to mix it up. Explore and find many options you like!

If we're not doing something we like, where's the benefit? Are we so compelled to look a certain way that we're willing to force ourselves to do things we don't like?

If we don't appreciate the journey, how can we appreciate the end when we reach our goals?

There can be struggle, sweat and hard work in a workout, but the work is always worth the reward, and the rewards last way beyond the actual workout itself. The rewards pay off time and time again.

The work is worth it. Always!

Challenge:
Using the resources available to you – books, the Internet, mobile applications and such – find three exercises that you are able to do, and are physically challenging. Practice each of those three exercises for one minute each, taking a 15 second pause between. Do three rounds of this activity. Take a one-minute break, and then go for a 20-minute walk.

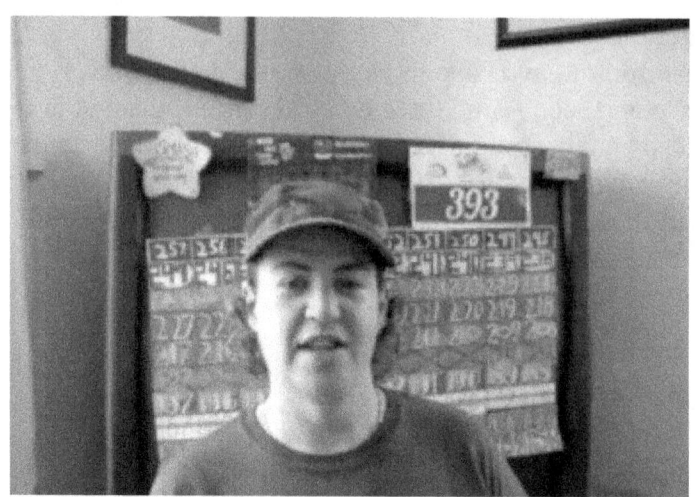

Reason #31 – <u>To stay sober and stay off alcohol</u>
Recorded on June 3, 2013

I'd love to say that in this journey I've been cured of my addictions. However, recovery has shown me that addiction isn't something that goes away. It's something we learn to live with.

From the video for this reason:
This is all a journey, and it's a lifestyle. It's about taking it one day at a time…incidents happen, we all make mistakes.

I'm so grateful for my clean time and sobriety. While working on this project, I had an inkling that I was going to have to get clean (stay off drugs) and sober (stay off alcohol) to really believe what I was saying and have the integrity to back it up. The choice was either to continue to convince myself that I was "sober" and could legitimately talk about this stuff, or to be truly honest, brave, and LIVE it.

Thankfully, the latter happened, and I'm so grateful for every day that I get to be clean and sober. Now, the feelings I used to have when I'd use drugs or get drunk are made real and authentic by doing things that I love every day. I don't have to put harmful substances into my body in order to feel good anymore – now, I feel elated every time I practice yoga, pray, work on my recovery, and when I skate. During an evening skate I took while writing this book, I saw a shooting star and was so touched. It was beautiful, and I didn't have the chance to make a wish because I was just staring at it, fully immersed in the present moment. After it was gone, I wondered what I would wish for, and I realized that my wish had already come true.

I'm clean and sober, and that is a wish granted for every moment I get to be alive to experience it. The feelings are so real, and even the bad ones are better than the emptiness I felt when I was using.

Very much like eating overly indulgent foods in vast quantities all the time, constantly getting high or drunk always led to regret and sickness. I had enough of it, and I'm so thankful that I gave up alcohol when I did (my last drink was on December 31st, 2008). It's not a part of my life anymore. It took a bit longer to finally admit I had a substance problem, but I finally admitted it and stopped using drugs (that was on September 24th, 2015). I'm working a program, and today, I'm clean and sober.

My authentic self is the best version of me, and the best version of me is clean and sober!

As a bonus, this is a great quote from the video for this reason:
I might not be ripped, but I'm strong. I might not be thin, but I am fit. I am not perfect, but I sure as hell work my ass off to be my best. There's a lot to be said for that.

Finally, here's a great "before" picture that I share in the video!

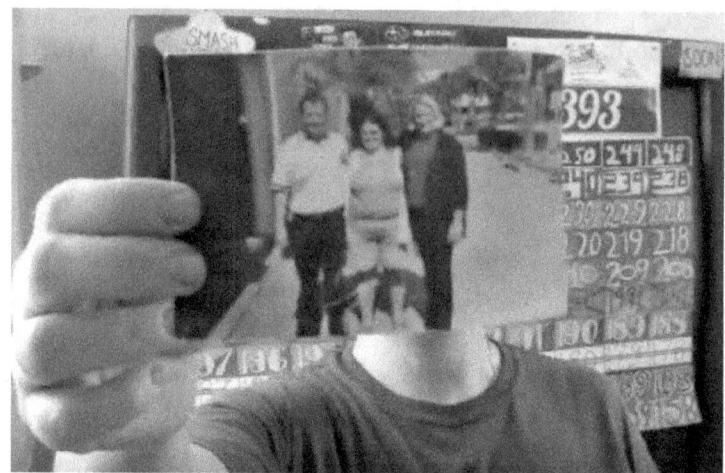

That's me in the center!

Questions:
Has addiction affected your life?
What helps you stay on point and out of trouble?
What's an obsession and/or compulsion you'd like to get help with?

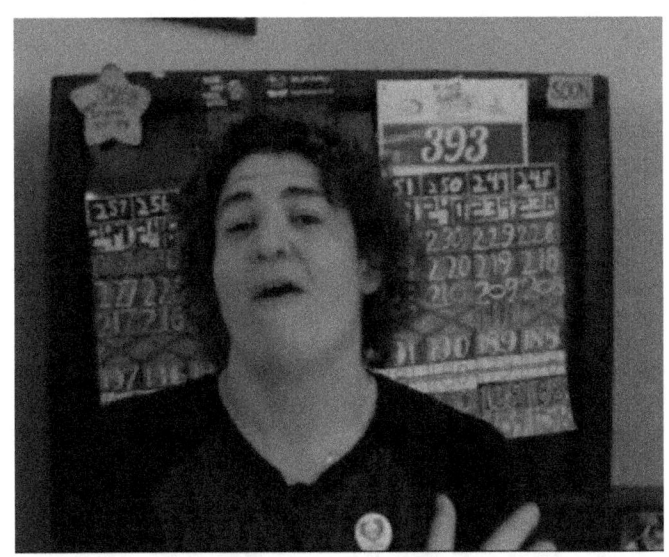

Reason #32 – <u>To feel like a boss when I touch my arms</u>
Recorded on June 4, 2013

From the video for this reason:
*I feel like a boss when I touch my arms **now.***

When I wrote the reasons, I wanted to have strong, sculpted muscles, especially my arms (since they're so visible). When I shot the reason, though I still wanted to keep shredding body fat, I was already feeling like a boss when I touched my arms (in the video, I kept touching my arm)! Now, I feel proud for what I'm capable of, how strong I am, and how my muscles look and feel. I *do* feel like a boss when I touch my arms! I love touching my arms now!

I'm super happy and proud of the results that have come from hard work! My arms are strong, toned and defined. My entire body is functional and strong, thanks to good nutrition, consistent strength training, cardiovascular exercise, and lots of yoga!

I have lots of reasons to wear sleeveless shirts and tank tops!

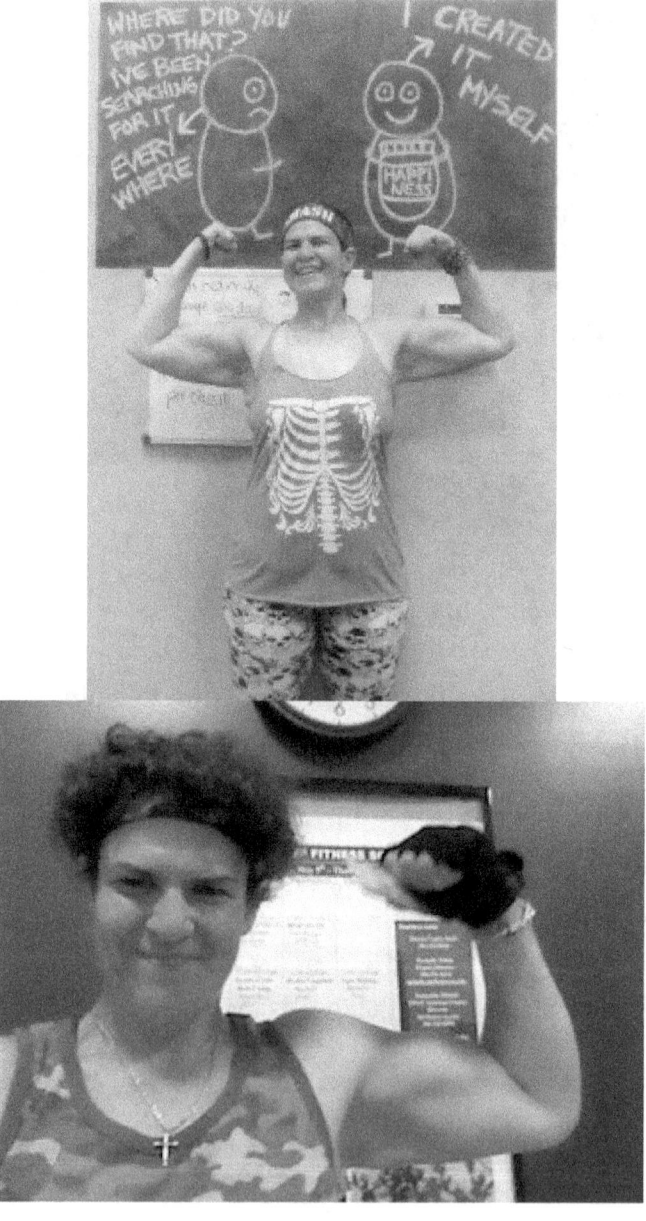

Beast feeling? Hell yeah!!

Activity:
Find an old t-shirt that you can use for a creative project. If you don't like the front graphic, turn the shirt inside out. Cut off the sleeves, and using fabric paint, write an inspirational quote or paint unique artwork on the back. Use references – the Internet is super helpful (hint hint...especially Pinterest!)

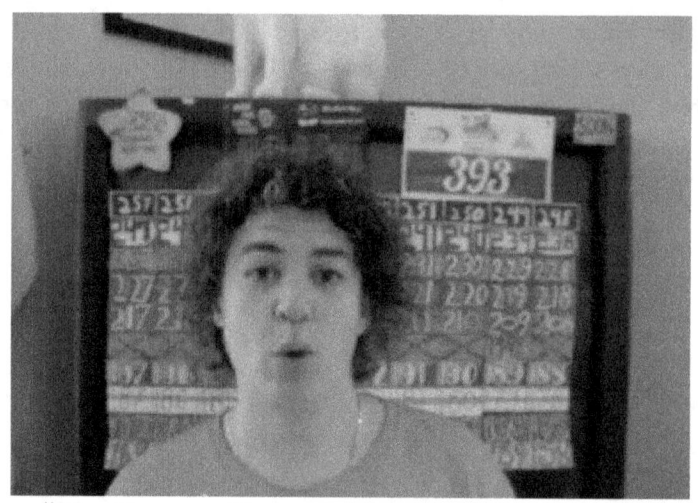

Reason #33 – <u>Because I know I don't need to change, and I won't change</u>
Recorded on June 5, 2013

We often compare ourselves to our "best" and past selves. While everything isn't perfect, we are here, and this is now. As long as we're doing the best we can, that's the most we can ask of ourselves.

Even when I hit my goal weight, I wanted to change my body – put on more muscle, add more body fat to tighten my loose skin, and bulk up because I was looking too lean, fill out my hips so I could be more effective in derby...the list goes on and on.

When I started this journey, I valued myself as a person and knew I could grow to learn to love myself (or at least learn to accept myself). During my transition into a healthy lifestyle, I learned to adapt, deal with setbacks (self-imposed and the lovely surprises life throws my way), and find where I needed to slow down, and where I could step it up. When I hit my goal, I was so accustomed to focusing on weight loss and I didn't give myself a moment to really bask in what I had accomplished.

The lesson here is that there will always be opportunities to grow, and it's important to first accept where we are and *who* we are before we go trying to change ourselves.

We all have flaws. It's actually our flaws that make us remarkable, if we can do something positive with them. Flaws provide amazing opportunities for growth! For instance, being an addict – because I am a recovering addict, I speak a language that many addicts speak, whether they're recovering and want to stay clean, or if they're active in their addiction and want to take steps toward recovery. Either way, being a recovering addict is a great quality because SO many people are affected by addiction, and I can help them by being dedicated in my recovery. I can take action to show them how it's done. I am certainly not perfect, but I can keep getting better, every single day. There are no perfect people. Those we hold in such high regard have tremendous flaws, just like the rest of us. When we've had an experience and find success, we have an obligation to share from the other side.

We have to soldier through the darkness to see the light, and only the light chasers can authentically speak about the journey out of darkness.

While amazing things happen in our lives, we come to accept that we've always been the same person. We don't have to change, and we can just keep growing!

Assignment:
Find your high school yearbook and read through the comments that your friends wrote. Journal about how this made you feel back then, and how you feel now.

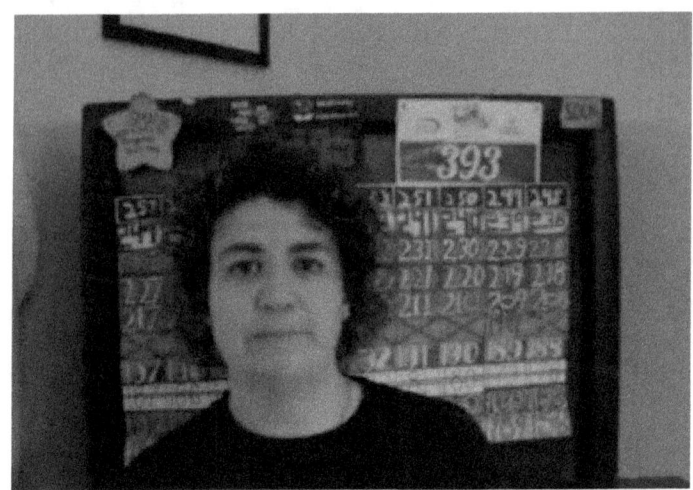

Reason #34 – <u>To better understand what I want</u>
Recorded on June 6, 2013

Hard experiences give rise to finding gratitude. When we're not having our way or getting what we want, we have the opportunity to be grateful for what we already have.

From the video for this reason:
What I wanted two years ago was a half-gallon of ice cream, and to be complacent... and now, instead of buying all the ice cream and the crap, I'd much rather register for Run for Your Lives, or get ready for a triathlon, or wanting somebody that's right for me, that deserves me. Thank goodness for this experience, because it definitely shapes things better, and what we want shapes how we're going to pursue it. Here's to the continual pursuit of good things that I want.

Desire can be fueled by the mind's ego, or the heart's wishes. When we listen to our hearts, our decisions are based in love. When we listen to the ego, we're slaves to insatiable desire. The heart is much wiser.

How do we know the difference?

The heart is always happy to pursue its wishes. The ego is never happy; it's only temporarily satisfied until it creates another burning desire.

96

The heart feels settled when we appreciate; the ego is pleased when we compete.

Listen to the heart. It speaks in stillness. Quiet the mind, and feel, sense, and tune in to the greater good. Forget the ego. It's a wailing child and is never at peace. Find peace by trusting your heart's guidance.

Assignment:
Review your goals in your notebook, your weekly plan, and your vision board. Are you working your plan? Add another goal if it's happening easily, modify if it's too much, and adjust as needed. Review your goals and your plans for action on a weekly basis, and again every month.

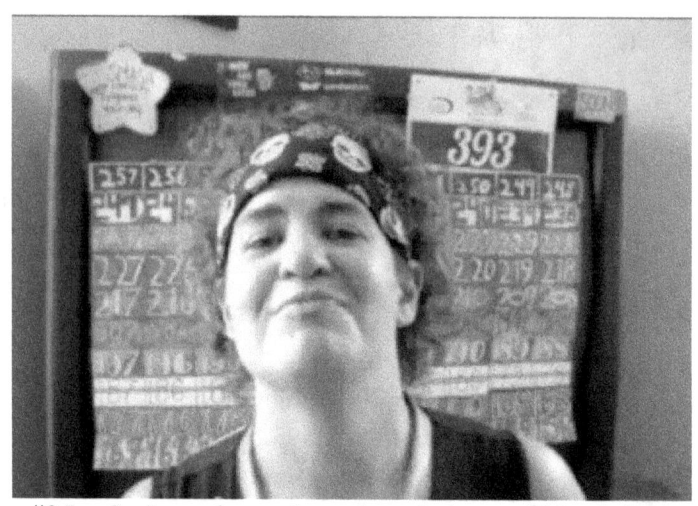

Reason #35 – <u>So I can brag about it and show off (and that's okay!)</u>
Recorded on June 7, 2013

This reason is all about celebrating accomplishments! Bragging is often considered comparative, but as the saying goes, beauty is in the eye of the beholder. It can also be used as a tool to share the spotlight, to cast the light of hope onto others, to encourage and empower them to reach their goals.

We can ALL win. Life *should* be a win-win. There's one earth and over 7 billion of us. Let's do this together, to raise each other up instead of tear each other down.

Brag, but do it to raise people up. Share the love. We've got so much to give and it comes from an infinite source of good. Draw from it and keep spreading it all around. It comes back, over and over, more of it flows in than we put out, if we spread it for the sake of uplifting, not competing or comparing.

To live as champions and raise champions, THAT is what it's all about!

Activity:

A brag book has many uses – applying for a job, asking for a raise, networking, fundraising, and overall esteem-building! Compile a brag book, first by reviewing your previous assignments and notes, and make a list of as many things you can think of that you've accomplished. Then, write a master letter, asking your associates, business partners, teammates, leaders, mentors, family members and community contacts, asking them to give you a character statement to add to your brag book. Then, email or send out the letter. Add their responses to your brag book. Also, include any letters of commendation, performance reviews and positive accolades you've received. Include anything you'd like – certificates of achievement, pictures and stories from community events, races, Most Valuable Player awards – whatever you'd like!

Bonus:

Make this a group activity and have a bragging crew participate with you! As you all work on your brag books, tell stories about experiences you've had that made you proud, compliment one another, and share stories about your friends that made you proud of them. Add entries in each other's brag books!

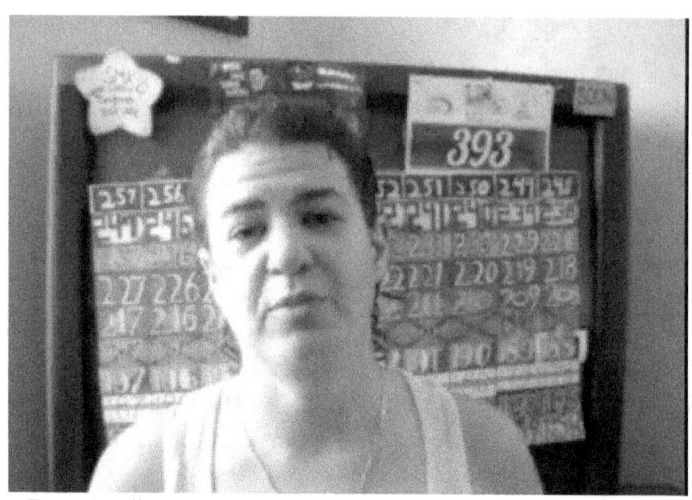

Reason #36 —<u>To appreciate hunger versus boredom</u>
Recorded on June 10, 2013
Weight: 188 pounds

Having a plan, a schedule, and structure are great ways to stay on track. If I have my meals planned and prepared, I'm then free to utilize my time and efforts on better things instead of wondering what I "want" to eat.

Eating is another natural escape to fall into, just like any other activity that can be used excessively – drinking, using drugs and medications, sex, even exercise – and it's smart to be mindful of what we're eating as well as how we're eating.

Logging meals and moods helps recognize patterns. When we can see patterns, we can come up with a plan to optimize our habits.

It's both fortunate and unfortunate that we cannot give up food altogether. We can abstain from many harmful and excessive habits, and eating is something that we can moderate and learn to utilize wisely.

I used to use food for every mood. Eating was a celebration, a coping strategy, an escape, a punishment (for myself, and when I was angry at others), a way to deal with sadness, depression, anxiety and fear. For any reason under the sun, I can find something to motivate me to eat. Even now, I still think about food quite often. It is still an everyday challenge to moderate my nutrition, and to take it easy on myself when I make a mistake and have too much. Sometimes, I go overboard. There are some things that I've eliminated altogether (candy bars, gummy bears and ice cream), and some things I am just not ready to walk away from (meat, carbonated water, Doritos – GOD how I love Doritos).

Failing is easy. Gaining weight is easy. Going back to old bad habits – see where this is going?

Taking steps back is just part of the journey. Getting back up and starting again, whenever it happens, is what helps build long-term results. Giving in to temptation now and then is fine. As long as we get back on track again, we'll keep thriving!

A healthy lifestyle means learning how to live well in every facet of our lives, and eating is a huge part of it. So, eat well, eat often, and eat to perform!

Assignment:
Log your meals and moods for the next week. Look for patterns. Create an action plan if you notice any harmful or disturbing habits. When logging, it doesn't have to be fancy and it doesn't have to be calorie-counting. Just note what you've eaten, how much, the time of day, and how you felt before, during and after. This will help create a new habit, and to recognize patterns!

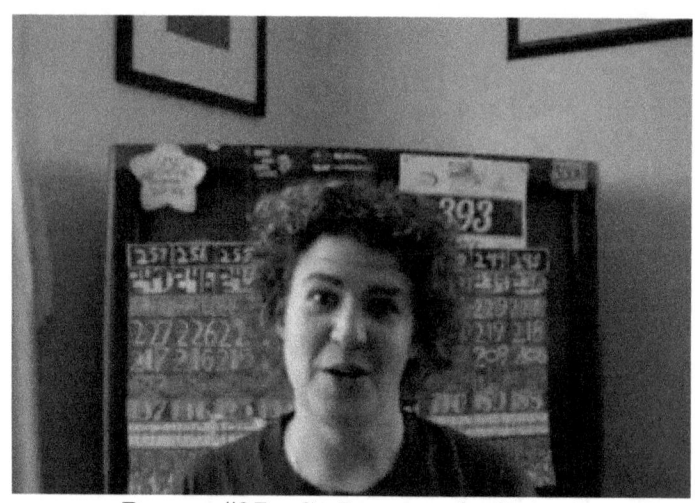

Reason #37 – <u>So I can go skydiving!</u>
Recorded on June 11, 2013
Weight: 185 pounds

I have wanted to go skydiving for as long as I have had conscious memory. It's been in my mind ever since I've seen airplanes, and without even knowing that it could be done, I wanted to skydive!

The first time I ever went to go do it, I was over the weight limit. Pissed about being rejected and angry at myself for not losing enough weight to do it, of course I did what any addict does – I fell right back into my addiction. I ate to fill that void. The 25 pounds I lost came right back and brought some friends.

Fifteen years after that first attempt, I finally did it! I lost the excess fat I'd been carrying on my body, and I rewarded myself with a skydiving voucher!

It was unlike anything I could have imagined, and the thrill of completely surrendering and relinquishing control was fantastic! Skydiving stripped away fear. I figured if I was to go, what better way than by witnessing God's earth, coming right at me at over 120 miles an hour?

There was this moment right before my tandem person pulled the ripcord that we got super narrow and fell deeper and more quickly right before the chute opened...it was incredible. Then, everything was in slow motion. The blue-green tones of the landscape focused in from a blur to more defined swaths of color. The ground went from racing toward me to patiently waiting for me. My body went from shooting like a bullet, narrow in front and wider in the back (because of our position, my body was in a type of U-shape), to hanging lazily, like the baby being pulled up from its overalls for observation by the Terminator in *Terminator 2*.

That experience will be with me for the rest of my life. As soon as we hit the ground, I was ready to do it all over again!

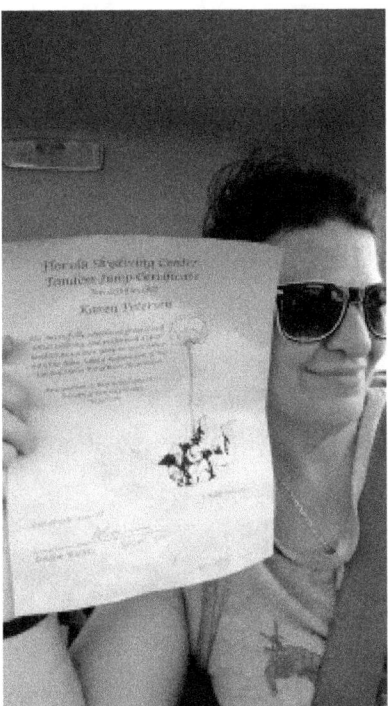
Post-jump shot!

Like so many things in life, there was SO much anticipation leading up to it! The event itself was so short-lived yet thrilling, and TOTALLY worth the work and time to earn it!

What a thrill! I can't wait to do it again!

Questions:
What is something you've been holding off on doing?
What has held you back from doing it?
How will you make that happen?

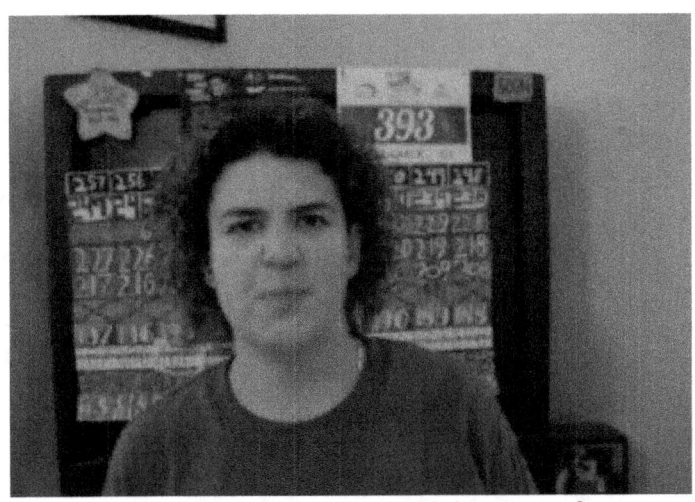

Reason #38 – <u>To be a much better surfer</u>
Recorded on June 17, 2013

From the video for this reason:
That moment, when I stood up on the board, and I surfed and got back into the water, I felt the presence of a friend of mine who passed away a few years ago, and then I felt God. Something happened. Everything opened and truth was revealed to me, and it was 'this is good and you should do it.'

That moment happened when I was over 250 pounds, and it was an astounding and stellar moment for me. Surfing is HARD. It's so hard; it requires a lot of core strength, upper body strength, and endurance. I tried and tried, and then finally one evening right before sundown, I popped up on the board and rode a wave. It was a moment I'll never forget, and every moment I was in the water after that was like chasing that initial feeling.

Surfing encouraged me to keep trimming down on my body fat, as the selections of boards are vast for folks under 300 pounds – though there are plenty of choices out there for full-figured folks!

Assignment:
Go to a sporting goods store or the sports supply section of a department store. Browse the selection of items and consider different activities, sports and hobbies that interest you. Ask the staff about the equipment, and imagine buying yourself something when you hit a milestone. Take a picture of it, put it on layaway, start saving and set a date on your calendar as the day you plan to reach your goal. Journal about the experience, noting what got you interested in that activity, how it made you feel when you went to the store, and what you're planning to do in order to make it happen.

Then, when you've reached that milestone, buy yourself that gift!

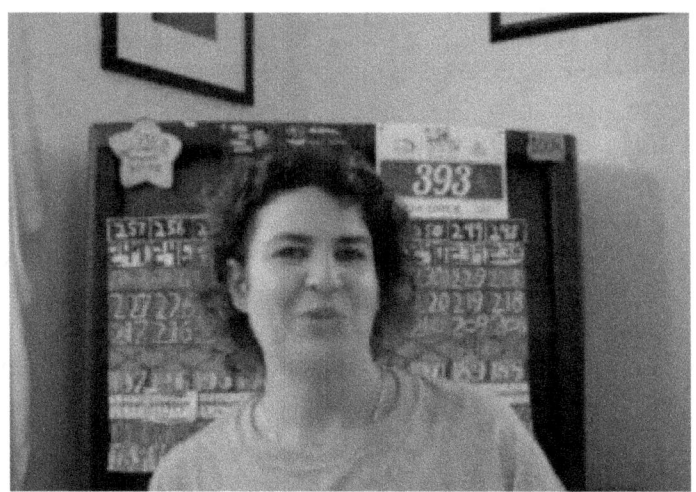

Reason #39 – <u>So I will be even hotter at my 20-year reunion</u>
Recorded on June 18, 2013
Weight: 186 pounds

Fitness had been quite elusive to me for most of my life, except for a few years during my most seminal physical and emotional growth – early teen years. I was "fat kid" for quite some time, and then I went through growth spurts and was involved in various athletic activities. I then reverted to unhealthy eating habits and stopped exercising. There was rarely ever a balance, ever.

When this list was written, I felt like I had a lot to prove. I cared what people thought and I judged myself harshly.

Now, I know better. I can't control people's thoughts, and their thoughts hold no bearing on my value. I knew these concepts for a very long time, and it has taken a lifetime to embrace them. Thankfully, this transition gave me great perspective, awareness, and improved self-worth.

I may or may not go to my 20-year reunion, and however it plays out, I'm proud of where I am today and what I've done to get here!

Activity:
Plan a get-together with people you enjoy being around, and make it something fun, interactive and engaging. Try throwing a game night, a movie marathon, watching a full season of a show, having a group dinner, brunch or holiday party on a non-holiday date! Encourage folks to dress up, to their comfort level. As the host, plan to dress well, with accessories and anything that makes you look and feel great. This activity is a great way to bring folks together, to take pictures and create memories! It's also designed to get you in the habit of sharing your experience with people you care about, and to look and feel good while you do it!

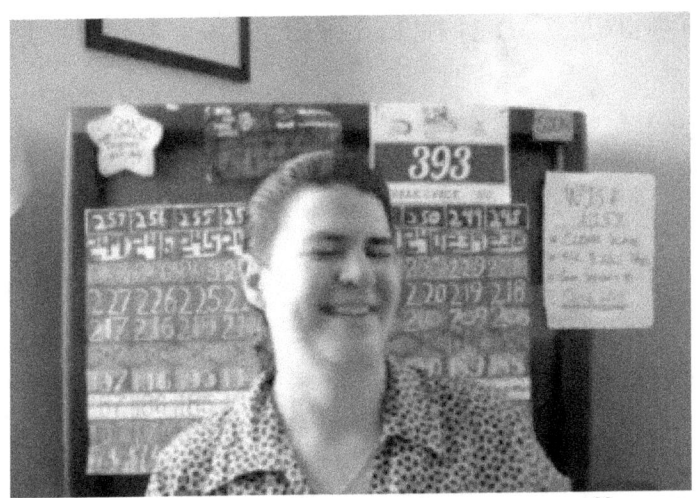

Reason #40 – <u>To try more crazy sex stuff</u>
Recorded on June 19, 2013

Sex is a great thing! It is an integral part of any intimate, romantic, committed relationship. Though I don't regret what prompted this reason and the actions that led up to this video, I've learned a LOT in the process about who I am and the importance of being honest with myself.

Freedom is an amazing thing. Now that I'm free from substance abuse, free from a sedentary, self-destructive lifestyle, isolation, and panic attacks, I'm ready for bigger and more amazing things.

I would like to get married. I do want a wife and to have the Happily Ever After.

Most importantly, I also want to be at peace with myself, to enjoy my own company without feeling compelled to take care of another person. I want to share my life with someone who can appreciate wholeness, because she herself is whole.

She'll find me; I'm going to let her come to me, instead of seek and chase her down. She'll come to me when I'm ready, and whenever that happens, who knows?

It's all on God's time. Only He knows what's best for me.

Assignment:
Take 20 minutes and write out a fantasy you've been holding onto for a while. Let it out. This is for you – no one is judging you and you don't have to share it. If you do want to share it, go ahead! That's what friends and partners are for! Without thinking, judging or feeling ashamed of yourself, write it all out, every dirty detail. Be creative and unabashed! There's no shame in fantasies. Allow yourself to release it, and whether it happens or not, just allow yourself to express your deep desires!

On a personal note:
I think it's pretty clear where I stand...after all, the reason states "*more crazy sex stuff.*" My fantasy is something I've wanted for a very, *very* long time. It's something I've wanted deeply in every relationship I've had, and (as of this writing), I have yet to experience it.

My fantasy is to experience love-making.

So, when I invite you to express your deep desires, aim high. Go for something you've always wanted. There are no taboos here. You'd be amazed what's "crazy" for someone is actually quite pedestrian for another. No judgment. Let your mind and creativity go totally free. No restraints (or, feel free to add in restraints in your fantasy, if that's what you're looking for)! This isn't about what other people consider "normal" or "civilized". It's *sex*! Sex is **anything** but civilized, clean and dignified. There's a reason we do it in privacy!

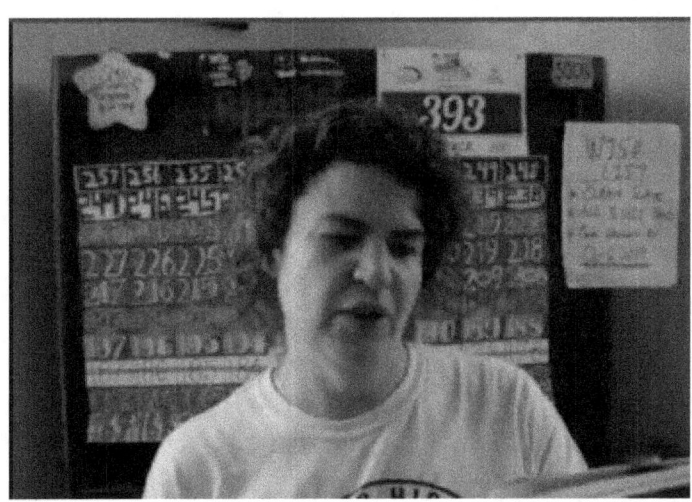

Reason #41 - <u>To feel the awesomeness of a mechanically sound body</u>
Recorded on June 20, 2013
Weight: 183 pounds

A mechanically sound body is a remarkable thing! I still marvel at how easy it is to get up off the toilet as a fit person; I remember having to brace the tub and sink to lift myself up for years. Now, I just stand up! Whenever I get up off the floor, now it happens so easily and naturally! There's not as much popping and cracking, no groaning and moaning from the effort. I'm so thankful that my body is functioning properly, that my muscles are strong, that my core gives me so much stability, and that I can look in the mirror and see my muscles that I've worked so hard for.

When it gets hard, I think about what it was like before. Being fit is recent, and my mind still thinks the same thoughts it did when I was nearly 300 pounds. Of course it does – I spent the majority of my life in an obese body.

When we tap back into those feelings while working toward a goal, we're armed with resources to continue onward when the going gets tough. Momentum is easy in the beginning; we have luck working on our side. When we get in the thick of it, that's when the challenge really begins.

In business, we get to the top, and our competition is seeking our position. Sometimes they may even take it. It's the same with fitness, except our competition is within ourselves, against that past self creeping in with its old thinking and old habits. Every day we must strive to do better than our former selves did, if we want to stay on top of our goals.

There's no comfort zone.

Questions:
How will you benefit from having a fitter body?
What tasks are a physical challenge for you?
How would you like to improve physically?

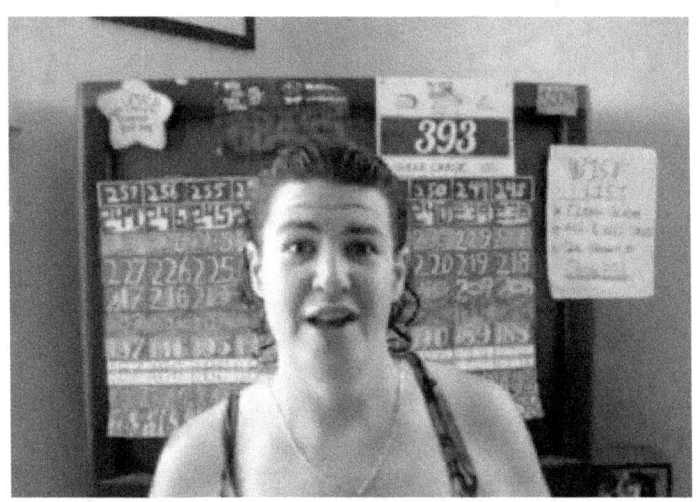

Reason #42 – <u>To turn heads</u>
Recorded on June 22, 2013

I've heard the phrase "when you look good, you feel good" and in my wellness journey, I have definitely found this to be true. For my entire adult life, I had held myself back and played small in order to be unnoticed. I really couldn't get away with that, since I have such a big personality. It was the classic contrast of wanting to show up big as well as play small.

Now that I feel authentically confident, I get more positive attention. For a while, it took some getting used to, because I really didn't know how to handle it. When strangers gave compliments, I felt a bit affronted (especially if they came from men). Once I felt better about how I'd look at people – just to enjoy the aesthetic, without creating any kind of attachment and feeling; comfortable with just looking (instead of feeling guilty for enjoying the view) – then I was able to receive compliments more comfortably. It was a long time coming; I got stared at a LOT when I was a child, and when I was a young teen, I had very short hair (due to a horrible reaction I had to a hair product that was used to tame my naturally curly hair) and was often asked if I was a boy or a girl. Even now, from time to time, I still get the occasional "buddy" or "sir."

If I want to turn heads in a positive way, I have to see myself in a positive light. If folks think or see it differently, I don't have to change that. I'm secure in who I am and their opinions don't matter if they differ from my own. How I feel about myself, in the end, is what matters the most.

No one has the power to define us, no matter what.

Assignment:
Compliment three strangers today. Make it a sincere compliment; it must be heart-felt, and kind. It can be anyone, for anything – how colorful and bright someone's tattoos are, someone's style, thanking someone you see with veteran stickers on his or her car. Journal how each of these experiences made you feel, and how the people reacted.

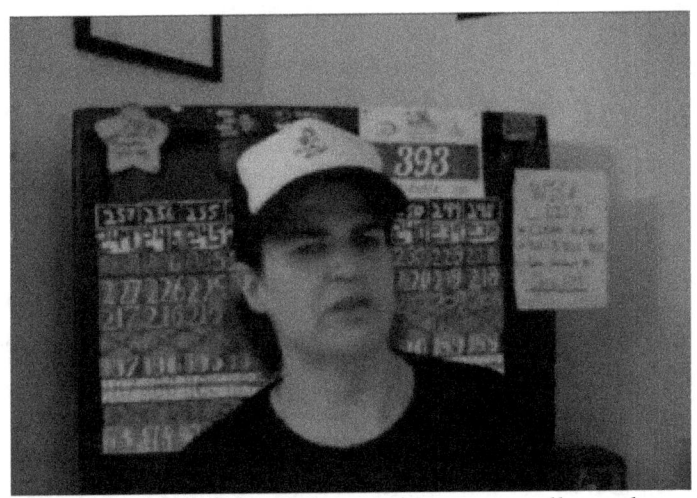

Reason #43 – <u>So I can wear out dogs on walks and runs</u>
Recorded on June 23, 2013

Dogs are amazing. Dog is also an anagram for God, and truly I see no coincidence there. The sweetest and kindest dogs have love in their eyes and are our best friends, and God is the very same.

I get so excited when I visit friends that have dogs – I LOVE dog-sitting and play time! It's like meeting a new friend and finding so much in common. I mean come on, we all really want the same thing – to give and receive love, to bring bright light into the world around us, to eat great food, to have someone hold us, play with us, run around and be free with us, and make us feel eternally young at heart. We want the best for people and we want the best for ourselves.

The phrase "the good die young" holds so true here. Dogs live a relatively short amount of time. They're meant to be adored and cherished in the little time we have with them. They enrich our world so much, and I sure hope that every person has the opportunity to, at least once, feel the unconditional love and happiness that dogs feel.

They're magnificent creatures!

I LOVE DOGS! I've always had cats, so I get my dog fix by volunteering at the local Humane Society. My favorite volunteer work is walking, running, and playing with dogs to get them exercised, out of their cages, and out in the open! The fresh air, attention and interaction light their beautiful faces up! It's also a great way to get exercise!

When I first started volunteering, the shelter staff told me about a former volunteer that was also a competitive track and field athlete. He spent hours running with dogs, helping them get their fix of attention, exercise and play time for the day. The staff and the dogs loved this volunteer, and he was able to help a lot of dogs because he had the endurance to work with a lot of them! This was great inspiration for me, and I wanted to get into the best shape possible so I could exercise with the dogs to help them work out as much energy as possible! A loved, exercised, and happy dog makes a well-behaved dog, and well-behaved dogs have a much better shot at finding forever homes.

I love that I get to use exercise as a reason to help save the lives of shelter dogs! The best part about this is that it's true! It works!

Activity:
Sign up to volunteer at a local animal shelter, and plan to spend a day (or, if you get hooked, at least one day per month) to interact with animals! Volunteering is great for the soul, and provides an excellent service to your community. If you have any animal allergies, plan a pet food drive with your friends and family!

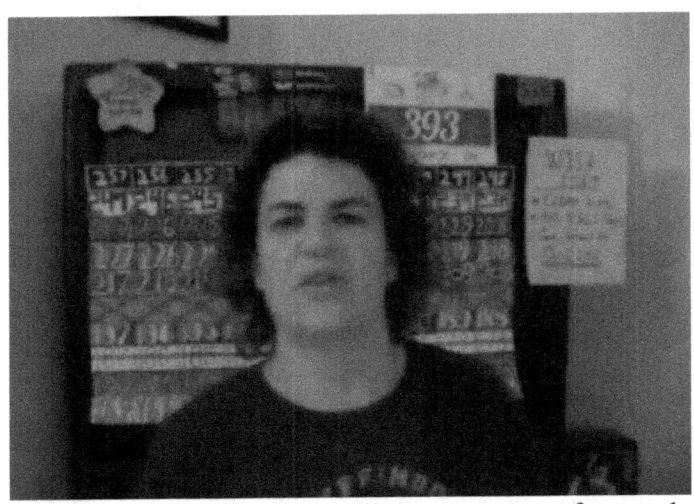

Reason #44 – <u>Because I will use my power for good</u>
Recorded on June 24, 2013
Weight: 183 pounds

What is the point of having power if it's not used it for good?

Having influence, being respected and living with heart's guidance affects others in a tremendously positive way! Success is a VERY powerful thing, and like popularity, it can raise people up. If we were to always act from love and with the intention of sharing our experiences, true change and positive personal evolution would become prolific.

There's PLENTY to go around! Good is abundant, non-competitive, and is meant to be shared!

When I wrote this reason, I was thinking about how some popular people (like kids in high school and some celebrities) act like total jerks when they have an audience. I had witnessed and experienced some bullying from popular kids, like I'm sure many of us have. When I wrote this, I imagined that people would treat me more favorably and that I would be liked more. I did find this to be true, but not because of external circumstances – it was because I was allowing them to treat me better. My vibe is way more positive, and that's appealing!

This journey has also humbled me. I thought I'd turn into an arrogant jerk if I ever got "attractive," giving me an inflated ego. Sometimes, I'd have moments where this was the case. Instead of practicing compassion for someone who would make a hurtful comment, I'd immediately think about a physical flaw and want to poke at the person who made the comment. Though I don't (usually, as far as I know) react, I'll admit that I still get the thoughts. However, I don't act on them. Being fit and healthy is a gift and creates a responsibility. I can't help but think of Uncle Ben's wise words to Peter Parker in Spiderman, "with great power comes great responsibility." This is also paraphrasing Voltaire (who really knew his stuff!).

Speaking of power, I've come to understand that power is a gift in mind, body and spirit. When I'm spiritually sound, I do good things for myself and for others. For instance, being spiritually sound helps me realize that I can do things daily to spread the light that a healthy spiritual life gives me. Little things, like telling people that I appreciate them, or handing out bottles of water and granola bars to people asking for money (I'd much rather give food than money) serve as a humble reminder that no matter the circumstances, I always can offer *something*. I don't have to be rich in order to brighten someone's day.

Questions:
How would you use influence?
What will you do when you reach your goals?
What is the title of your story now? What would you like it to be?

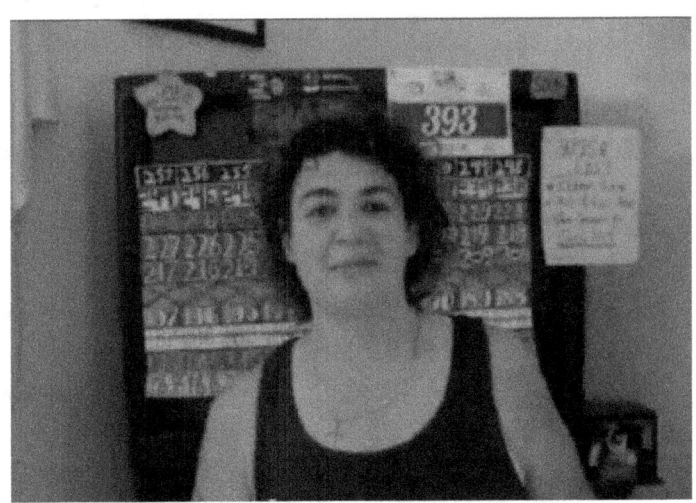

Reason #45 – <u>So I can have me time</u>
Recorded on June 25, 2013
Weight: 181 pounds

From the video for this reason:
By having my me-time, it gives me a chance to work on introspection, my meditation, my prayer, and doing whatever it takes to get me in a really good position to feel peace and function.

Getting "me time" means taking time to recharge our batteries, to meditate, pray, and do the things that we need to do on our own to come back to ourselves. Taking time for ourselves gives us the space and perspective to keep ourselves content, at peace, and healthy in mind, body and spirit.

We give so much of ourselves to others, and so we must bring focus and love back to ourselves. If we don't take care of ourselves and fill ourselves with love, it prohibits us from sharing it with others. We must have love in order to give it - our love and energy comes from within and we extend it outward! It's imperative to get charged so we can keep spreading our love and light!

Taking time for myself helps keep me calm, content, and better equipped to take on life's challenges, and just makes me a happier and healthier person overall. During my me time, I meditate, read, pray, listen to music, take a hot bubble bath by candlelight (a personal favorite), work out, or build a fire in my fire pit. I love watching a fire by myself; there's something about a fire pit that brings me calming, peaceful and very groovy vibes! Though I also enjoy sharing some of these activities with others, I love to do them by myself.

Activity:
Plan a pampering day. This is a day that you will set aside to treat yourself to a big reward! Schedule the date, save up for it, and when the day comes, indulge in this special day! Remember some of the suggested rewards (or come up with your own): a spa day, treating yourself to a massage, have someone take the kids for a long weekend and enjoy the home to yourself and/or with your partner, plan a trip and go – the list goes on and on! Cash in on that reward, and enjoy it!

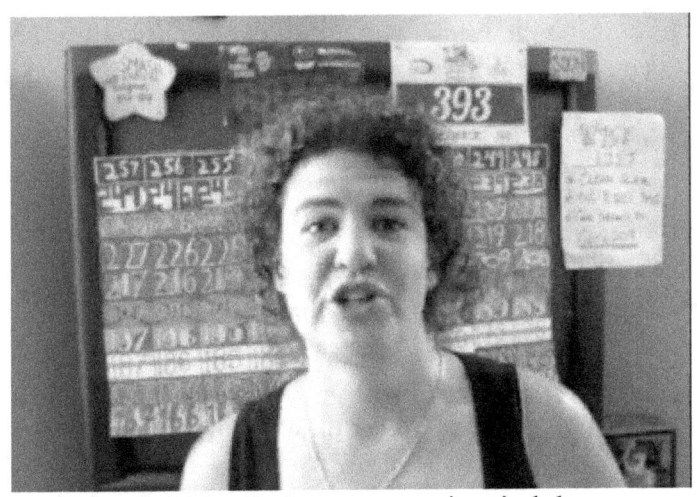

Reason #46 – <u>To better appreciate indulgence</u>
Recorded on June 26, 2013

It's important to know what things we can have in moderation, what things we have no control over, and also the habits we have in relation to these things. For instance, it's okay to have pancakes (I love pancakes!), and making them at home gives us more control of portion sizes than having them at a restaurant. Restaurant portions are typically WAY larger than normal serving sizes, and the nutritional information posted on their websites (and their menus, if available) is subject to the whims of the cooks and managers. I fall into a mindset thinking that they're just as mindful about portions as I am, and quite often, that's just not the case.

In the end, only we are in control. We know what a portion is, and how to control ourselves if we're given too much food. When eating out, our best bet is to ask for a to-go container when we order, so we can put at least half of it away when the food is brought to us. That's the key to moderation— knowing that we eat what's in front of us, it's how our brains are wired. We can arm ourselves with habits to counteract these tendencies.

Moderation with indulgences keeps us from going overboard. If I don't allow some pizza into my life when the cravings hit, then I'll go totally off the deep end and eat SO much pizza, either in one sitting, or go for several times during the week (sometimes even consecutive days) because I went from craving it to obsessing about it. Allowing a little bit of the things we crave keeps the demon at bay, and gives us back the control instead of let it control us.

Food is a tricky thing; we need food to survive, and yet those of us who struggle with moderation and making smart decisions fall prey to the seductive images, scents and temptations all around us.

There is hope, and it's created by arming ourselves with good habits, positive influences, and by knowing how to think about food, as well as what we can and what we just cannot have in our lives and in our bodies.

Good decisions come from an awareness of what we can and cannot have. By knowing ourselves, we're then smarter, wiser, and more capable of controlling ourselves. What we permit into our bodies and lives says a lot about how we feel, and sometimes we feel like we deserve a treat. Sometimes, it's just best to stick to the healthy stuff – especially after falling into old, bad habits again (goodness knows I can relate to that – especially when it comes to emotional eating)!

Balance, moderation, and most of all, knowing thyself. By knowing, we can make good decisions. Sometimes, that good decision is to just eat some pizza! Indulging in one or even two slices saves from eating a whole entire pizza in a single day!

Assignment:
Write in your journal about foods that you have absolutely no control over. Whether it's portion control, your go-to food of choice when you eat emotionally, or just plain sugar-laden candy and processed food, make a list of things that are huge trigger foods for you. Then, write about how you plan to remedy this. Can you still enjoy those foods if rationed out (for instance, portioning out a bag of Doritos instead of eating the whole thing in one sitting)? Spend at least 20 minutes on this assignment, and give it lots of thought and application!

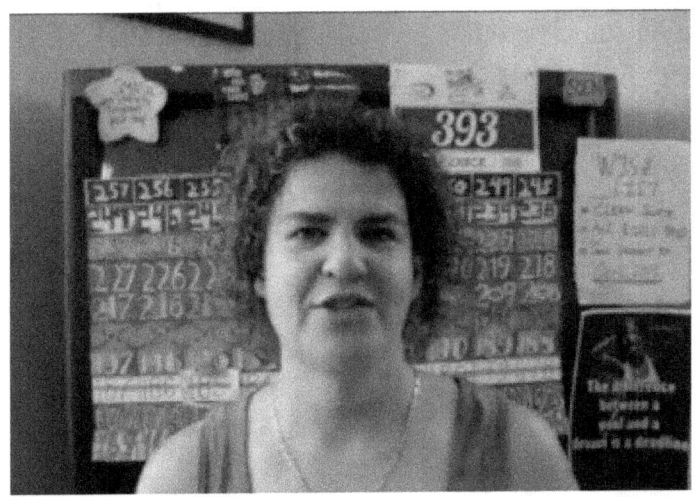

Reason #47 – <u>Because when I'm healthy, I'm less likely to procrastinate</u>
Recorded on July 8, 2013
Weight: 185 pounds

The blessing of a healthy mindset is that it is more than just "dieting" and "losing weight". It's a lifestyle change!

When we have a thought that requires action, it's best to take that action within five seconds of having that thought. Excuses and rationale are endless, and motivation and opportunities are fleeting. When there's a window to do something, just take action and DO it! That sets a habit in place, and it's a huge relief to just get that thing done instead of putting it off and worrying about it!

It can be simple, like putting on workout clothes to get ready for a workout. Instead of fixating on how hard a workout will be, just think about getting dressed. Break things down into steps, and then, before you know it, that seemingly impossible mountain will be conquered step-by-step!

Make small, realistic goals, and go through each moment one at a time. When feeling overwhelmed, just breathe. Focus on deep, mindful, full breaths, both in and out through your nose. Be in the moment, and

123

knock out one thing at a time. Setting small goals helps get LOTS done! When we get overwhelmed, it's easier to quit than to tackle a small goal. Be kind and pace yourself.

Questions:
What are some things you procrastinate on?
How can you remedy this?
What is something that you'd like to do that you've been putting off?

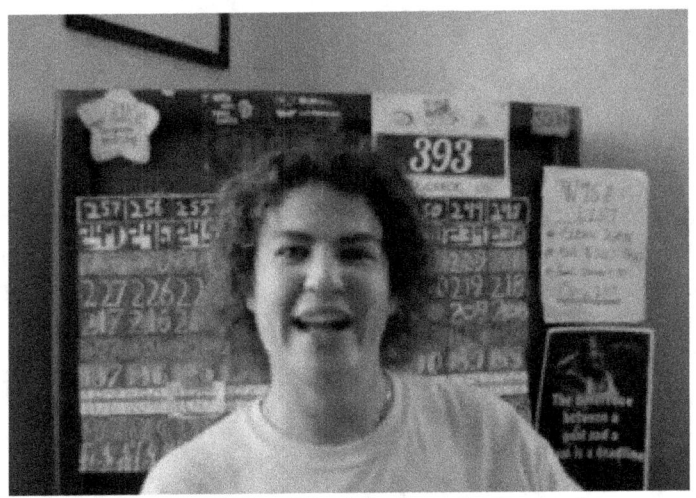

Reason #48 – <u>Working out feels good</u>
Recorded on July 10, 2013

Exercise gives us more energy, mental clarity, optimism, and often inspires a closer connection with our highest selves/Spiritual Source.

Working out is a challenge, and the rewards are incredibly beneficial! The euphoria of an endorphin rush is amazing!

A great way to develop a workout habit is creating the mindset. Break it down into small, manageable chunks (sound familiar?). Plan workouts into your weekly schedule. Mix it up to prevent boredom. Take a few group fitness classes, such as BodyPump, yoga classes, spinning, boxing, and whatever else strikes your interest! Read about various workouts and talk to friends who are fit to see what they are doing. Go with a group!

Humans have an innate tendency to go the easy and lazy route, and yet we feel energized, validated and happy when we complete a difficult task.

Imagine how wonderful the shift in mindset would be by incorporating regular workouts, and how you'll benefit from it!

Challenge:
Find a fitness center and sign up for a free class, or if you have a membership, take a class you've never taken. Bring a friend – the buddy system is amazing!

Extra bonus challenge:
Attend a roller derby practice! No skating experience required. Derby people come in every age, shape, size and socioeconomic status! Do some research and find a local league – Google and Facebook are great tools to help you with this. Contact the team and ask if they have loaner gear for newcomers. Or, take it a step further and attend a bout! Interact with the teams – you'll find that most roller derby folks are *very* friendly, helpful and enthusiastic! Give it a shot – it may very well become your next love (roller derby has special powers)!

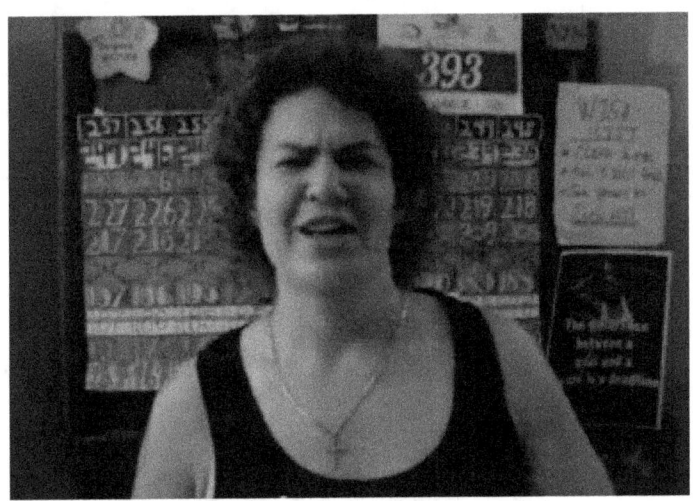

Reason #49 – <u>To retain my youth</u>
Recorded on July 11, 2013
Weight: 180 pounds

Too often in life we take ourselves too seriously, and we suffer because of it. Laugh at simple, little things. Have fun! By tapping into our inner child to keep things light-hearted, we feel and look younger, and our energy soars! When we think, feel and act young at heart and healthy, it shows!

This is a daily practice, so practice it every day!

We are born with curiosity, innocence, and the innate ability to love unconditionally. Over time, we learn negative things, create biases and build walls. Come back to the clean slate mentality of a child, and see things for how they truly are, not how we've been told to perceive and judge them.

Staying young at heart has been a secret to good health, so do these things as often as you can – laugh, sing, play, have fun, and keep things light-hearted! In the end, all the things we stress about, over time, become little things. Let them go. It's a simple principle, perhaps not easy, and definitely worth integrating into our lives. Keep it simple!

When I wrote this reason, I was feeling worn down and much older than I should for my age. I wanted to feel vivacious and optimistic again. Being youthful in heart, to me, means carrying joy instead of a heavy burden. This journey has lightened my load physically, mentally and emotionally. I find joy in activities such as skating, yoga, eating healthy and getting proper rest. Feeling happy, grateful and relieved has had remarkable results – I look and feel young again!

Activity:
Plan a funny movie or show night with friends and/or family. Invite them to bring healthy snacks, to wear silly outfits, and encourage funny accessories – masks, beads, ridiculous socks and such! Before the movie starts, ask each of your guests to share a funny story, joke, or quote. You're more than welcome to use the Internet for help with this! Take pictures and have them all write in the guest book you created in the activity for Reason #28. If you haven't created the guest book by now, have it ready in time for this activity! The guest book can be as simple as a notebook, or as ornate and decorated as you'd like it to be!

Bonus:
Watch a favorite movie from your childhood/youth!

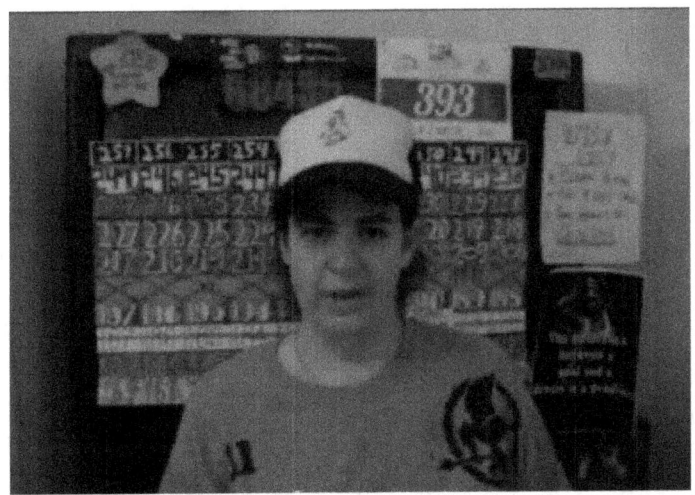

Reason #50 – <u>Because I love to move to kick-ass music</u>
Recorded on July 21, 2013

From the video for this reason:
You ever have one of those workouts where you just can't find you rhythm? You're like 5-10 minutes into your run and it isn't fun yet? Or, you've just busted your ass for the last half hour, hour, forty-five minutes and you just want to finish your workout? You're on your last legs, and you're done. And then, that song comes on, and BOOM! I got this shit, crank it up! Then the workout is great again, and next thing you know, you've found your second wind!

The right music brings a workout to the next level! Oftentimes, the right song will make us find that extra energy we've been holding in storage, and will get us to work harder, longer, and power through challenges in a workout!

Music can make work more bearable, a long drive way more enjoyable, and give us the extra energy we need for any activity. Music is a wonderful way to listen to stories and to appreciate amazing voices, melodies, harmonies, and great beats. There are all kinds of music for every possible mood, occasion and activity!

Music has been a huge love and passion of mine for as long as I can remember. I have many positive associations with music – singing in church and my elementary school choir, learning string instruments in middle school (and thus learning about classical music, which I love!), getting into dance and club music to fuel my workouts and attending concerts with friends (which creates amazing memories) – and I listen to music every day! Especially in the car. I have concerts in the car. I can't decide which is better – singing at the top of my lungs, or watching the reactions from the other drivers!

Assignment:
Create a workout playlist and listen to it throughout the day – before, during, and after your workout. You can mix it into your daily music, or listen to it by itself on the day you create it. Notice how it makes you feel when you're working out to it, and when you're doing other activities while listening. Journal your experience.

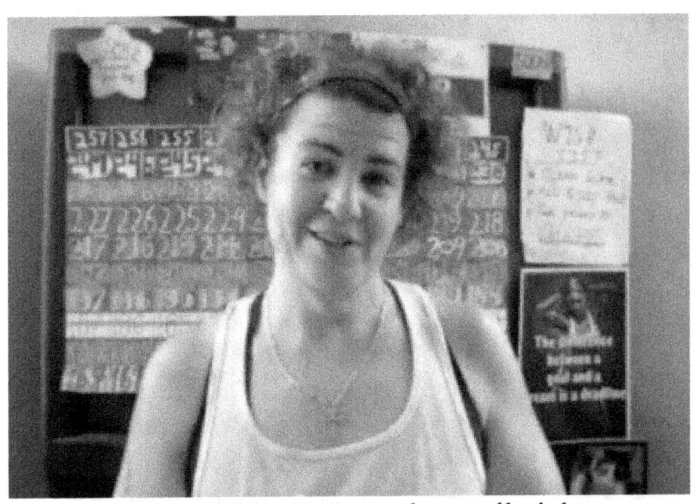

Reason #51 – <u>So I can dance all night</u>
Recorded on July 25, 2013

Dancing is great with a partner, a group, or just going at it solo. There have been many times that I've just broken down in dance at home, enjoying the music and moving along as I'm cleaning, doing housework, laundry and so on. It can be hard to get started (especially when it comes to folding laundry!) and then once I do, things get done!

Like many people, I get a bit hung up on how it should look, if I'm doing it "right", if my moves are good. However, dancing isn't about how it looks, it's about going with it and just enjoying the moment!

I'm that crazy girl at weddings that starts the dance-off and doesn't stop until the DJ is wrapping up…and even then I'm still moving! Regardless of how good, bad, fast or slow I'm going, I just love to dance. It's one of the best activities to vibrate a high frequency of energy, it produces endorphins, and damn it, it's just FUN!

Activity:
Put on upbeat music and dance as you do your housework, and dance and sing along! Don't half-ass your dancing – put your WHOLE body (and booty) into it! This is a great motivator to keep the house tidy!

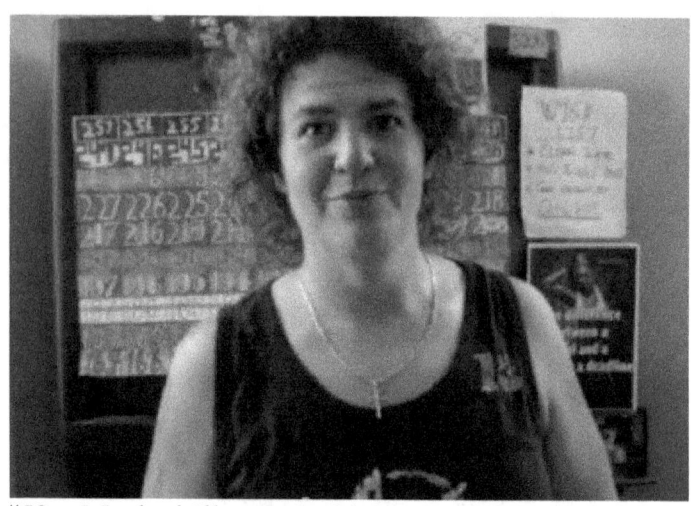

Reason #52 – <u>Maybe it'll stop the high school/middle school shit in my head when I pass a group of people</u>
Recorded on July 29th, 2013

In the past, I used to take things very personally. Whenever I'd hear a group of people laughing, I thought they were laughing at me – and sometimes, they were. This was exacerbated in middle school, which is when the number of students increased, just like the hormones (which made clique rivalries and bullying much worse). It lasted for years, even though I hoped it would subside as an adult. It didn't. Adults are just as bad – if not worse – than kids when it comes to cliques and taunting. I had some very personal experiences with this, but I've learned over time that it's not my problem if people are jerks. I'm not in control of how people behave, I'm only in control of how I react.

It's a natural human reaction to take things personally, especially if we're dealing with feelings of insecurity. We want to belong. We want to be liked.

That may not always be the case, and it's our task to love and accept ourselves. Not everybody will like us. We can't change that. When we learn to embrace who we are, the judgment of others has no bearing on our self-perception and self-acceptance. As we learn to accept ourselves, we naturally accept others, and this amazing dynamic occurs where we notice that they've accepted us, left us alone, or we're no longer affected by them.

Sometimes the thoughts still arise, sometimes we still get angry, and sometimes we want to react to what someone has said or done, and that's okay. It's what makes us human. We're flawed, we have egos, we have issues. As we live, we learn. We make mistakes, we take a few steps back, and then we move forward again and learn as we go.

Self-acceptance is one of the greatest gifts we can give ourselves as we live a healthy lifestyle, and it doesn't always have to be perfect. It is a daily habit and as we practice it daily, it becomes more natural!

Questions:
What makes you feel loved and accepted?
What are some qualities in others that annoy you?
How are you impacted by the judgment of others? Would you like to change that?

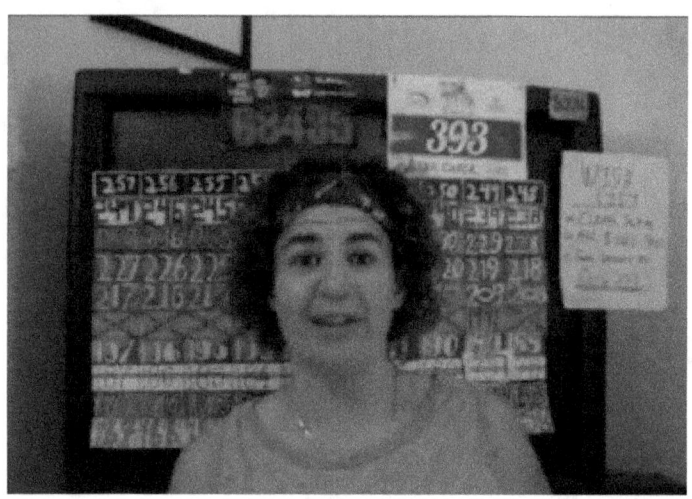

Reason #53 – <u>Because I want to do my damn boudoir pics</u>
Recorded on August 6, 2013
Weight: 179 pounds

This reason was inspired by friends who have shown me pictures that they had taken for their significant others. I was floored by how beautiful, sexy, and confident they looked in their pictures, and it gave me a new perspective on them. It also made me realize that I can do that as well – and for myself!

Some of the greatest moments in life come when we don't think, we just *do*. When I am photographed by a professional, I feel natural, playful, and hot. It's a hell of a lot of fun!

I keep giving the excuse that the photographer I had sought out flaked on me, but whatever the actual reason, I haven't gotten these photographs done yet. It's about damn time that I do it. I suppose a part of me is afraid that they'd be perceived as overly sexual, as I've been abstinent, waiting to fall in love again and commit to a relationship with someone who is on my level and inspires me to be amazing, but the reality is these are just for me. Just like I took on this project as an act of self-love, my boudoir pictures are also a present to myself.

So now I ask myself – what am I waiting for?

And to you – what are you waiting for?

Challenge:
Set the mood – light candles, put on music, and dress in something that makes you feel sexy (or forget the outfit altogether). I recommend doing this for yourself and by yourself, however if having your significant other with you helps, then have at it! Look at yourself in the mirror and tell yourself how sexy you are. Remind yourself that you are desirable. Look yourself in the eyes and say it until you feel it. It may happen quickly or it may take a while, so keep at it until you truly feel it. You may laugh, you may express a variety of emotions, and those are all good. Just allow yourself to look, feel and be totally natural. Authenticity is sexy! Then, reward yourself – a hot bubble bath is a great option! If you're doing this with a partner, surely you'll come up with something to do together! After you finish, journal about the experience. Note how you felt before, during and after.

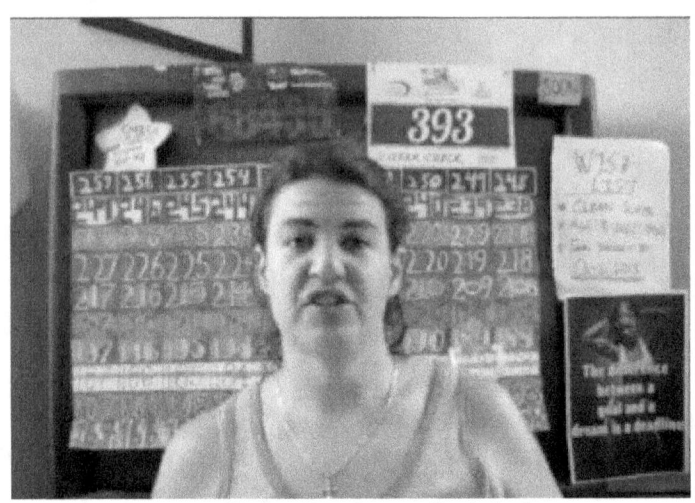

Reason #54 – <u>To sleep all night long</u>
Recorded on August 7, 2013

Healthy living has a great impact on our sleeping habits! It's remarkable how being healthy, eating well and getting enough exercise can give us the amazing blessing of great rest.

Proper sleep yields amazing benefits: stress and anger management, recharging, restoration, and relaxation. We work hard and need our rest to go at it strong the next day!

Isn't it interesting that fitness is a big contributor to a healthy lifestyle, and so is rest? Isn't it funny how we need to eat in order to lose weight?

It's not a magic formula, it's simply mathematics. Just as we need food to fuel our bodies, we need rest to restore ourselves for optimal performance.

I've had horrible sleep patterns over the years, especially when I wasn't taking care of myself. A reactive (not planned) schedule, overeating, physical activity avoidance, anxiety, depression and obsession impacted my sleep to the point that I later developed insomnia. That changed once I got healthier. At first, it was strange adjusting to a sleep pattern – I went from getting little sleep (like 2 hours or so) to sleeping up to 8-10 hours! That had an immensely favorable impact on my habits overall, especially interpersonal relations! I became much nicer once I got some rest! It also made choices easier for me – when we stress, we're likely to fall into bad habits.

These things seem like common sense, but what makes sense is often something we run away from. Even if they're not common practices for you, they can be. So again, keep it simple. Get your rest!

Assignment:
Review your weekly schedule and make any modifications needed, ensuring you've given yourself ample time for rest, recovery and sleep. Get very specific here, and log how much time you're spending on activity as well as recovery. For instance, are you using time intervals, like 50 minutes of work followed by 10 minutes of rest? Look into productivity resources, like time blocking. Then, develop strategies for how you'll implement these techniques into your daily schedule.

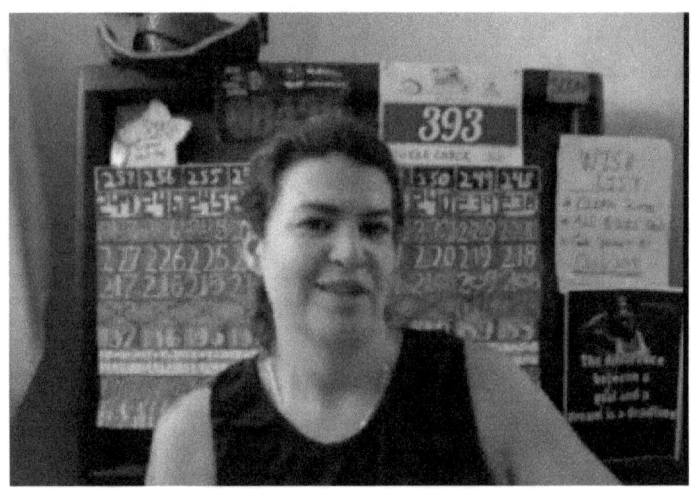

Reason #55 – <u>Solid poop schedule and a clean colon</u>
Recorded on August 19, 2013
Weight: 181 pounds

When I wrote this reason, I was dealing with serious gastrointestinal disturbances. I was under the care of two doctors for help with the physical and emotional symptoms that had affected my health. I was stressing myself out so badly that it was manifesting in my innards. My poop schedule was erratic, and the consistency was disgusting. My body was attacking itself and I felt horribly. Then, in turn, my stress rose.

Thankfully, with time and good habits, I've gotten myself in a good place with my health and my stress management. Sure, I still get upset, I still get angry, and I certainly still have anxiety, but my reactions are FAR different than when I wrote these reasons. As of the time of this writing, over a year has passed since I've had a panic attack, and I've been off medications for over a year as well.

We still have thoughts that influence us, but it's ultimately our actions that speak the loudest. We can be upset about something that happened, but if we go and make it our Facebook status update, and bitch and whine to people about it, then we're just feeding into it more and more. If, instead, we give it up in prayer and go on with our lives, and continue to practice good habits and take the right actions, then we've

138

honored what our highest self wants for us. We do the thing we keep telling ourselves we "should" do, and instead of wait for another Monday, or for specific conditions, we find that making the right choice here and now makes ALL the difference!

Taking action and thinking, feeling, and behaving like a good person has a tremendously positive effect on our overall happiness. When we're happy, we're less likely be stressed. Less stress means decreased illness. So, be happy! Your colon will thank you!

It's nice to feel great instead of feeling shitty!

Questions:
Is your digestive system healthy?
Do you find your body is on a steady elimination schedule?
How can you bring more peace into your life in order to stress less?

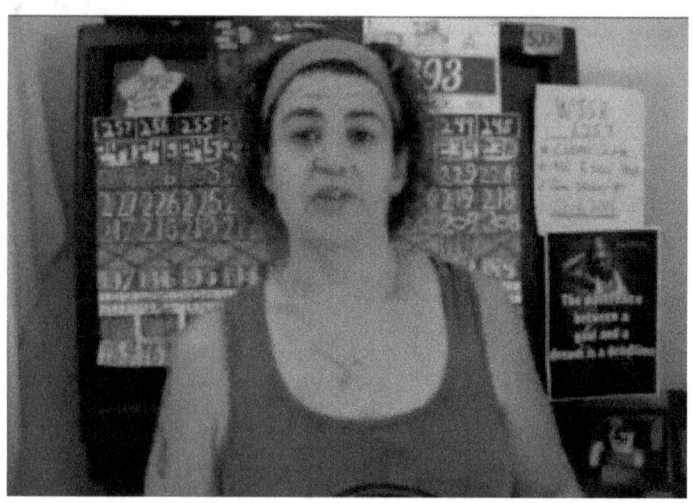

Reason #56 – <u>To improve my race times</u>
Recorded on August 21, 2013
Weight: 176 pounds

Races are a great reward for getting fit! Registering for a race is a reward itself, and on the day of the actual event, the energy and the vibe are fantastic! Themed races with obstacles are a LOT of fun, especially when running with a buddy or a team!

When I wrote this reason, I was thinking about running races, from 5K runs to the Disney Marathon. My first 5K race ever was a virtual race, and that was part of my training for my first live race – the Dash Down Greenville 5K in Dallas, TX. I'll never forget that race – it was during St. Patrick's Day weekend, and Greenville Avenue is a huge party-revelers destination, especially for St. Patrick's Day. As I approached the first drink stop, I heard another runner say "that's not water!" Turns out there were drink stops with green beer! At 8AM! I kept going until I hit an actual water stop, and once I finished the race, I enjoyed the complimentary green beer that each race participant was awarded at the end (this race was before I gave up drinking)!

This reason was written before I broke my ankle, and I had run several races before I broke my ankle from skating. But since then, I've switched from running to roller skating for my go-to endurance activity. It's a happy switch, because I actually abhorred running! Funny thing – I don't like running because it bothers my bionic ankle, but I love to skate...which is how I broke my ankle! It's a challenge, and one that I'm happy to take on. Every time I gear up, I think about where I started, and how far I've come. I wasn't a good skater for a long time. I've put a lot of time and mileage on my skates, and that's helped my skills and my confidence.

Skating can be very meditative and calming; it's another way to reach higher consciousness and find peace in the present moment. It requires coordination and awareness. When I skate, I must stay focused, aware of my surroundings, and in touch with what's going on around me. It's a great way to get out of my busy mind!

Tracking my mileage and pace (I use the Endomondo app) keeps me accountable and keeps me pushing myself to grow! Measuring progress is a great way to stay motivated and to keep stepping it up! Having goals keeps my training from getting boring, and when I mix it up, it's always interesting!

Activity:
Get a group together and find a race to do as a team. Pick a day close to day of the race and have a shirt-making party. Plan for race day, decorate shirts, and plan a post-race celebration! Shirts can be hand-painted, designed, or your group can work with a t-shirt printing company to create team shirts. On race day, take lots of pictures and enjoy the event – there's so much going on at races! Interact with the participants and share stories. Most of all, have fun!

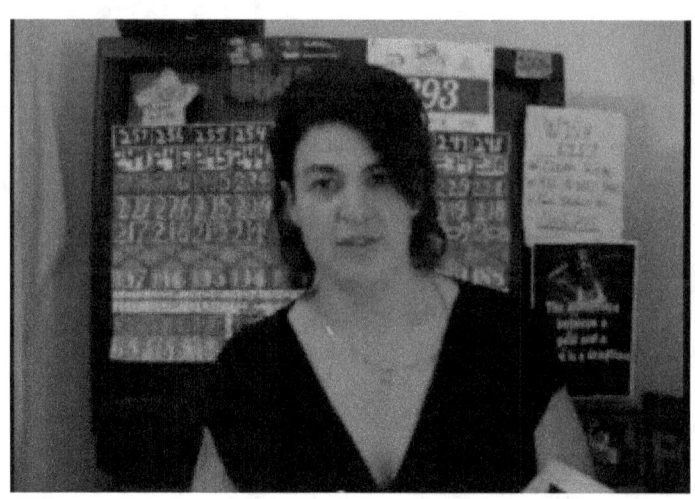

Reason #57 – <u>To run the Disney Half in November</u>
Recorded on August 21, 2013
Weight: 174 pounds

When I wrote this reason, I was inspired by several friends who had run the Disney Marathon and by various folks in the racing community who had told me that the Disney races are among the best in the world. Back when I wrote this reason, I was all fired up to start running races again, and I wanted to knock a marathon off of my bucket list.

I can gladly say that I've knocked it off, and not in a way I had originally intended!

I've skated 30+ mile distances several times now, and there are skating races that I'm excited to take part in! The training routine is challenging and it is fantastic motivation for me to keep my fitness routine going strong. Skating a race is way more appealing to me now than running was!

Skating national landmarks has been fun (albeit risky...which perhaps is what added to the fun factor!), and I wonder if, one day, I'll try skating around Disney World!

Questions:
What are some of your bucket list items?
How do you plan to do these activities?
What's holding you back from doing them now?

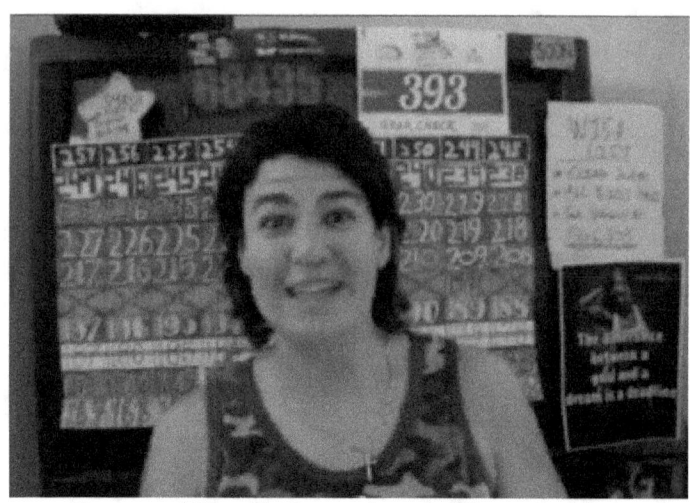

Reason #58 – <u>So I can do an effing triathlon</u>
Recorded on August 22, 2013
Weight: 174 pounds

A triathlon is WAY more appealing to me than the other races I'd considered before, even with the running component…which, of course, comes at the end of the race. The run, for me, would be the most arduous component of the triathlon, because again, I'm just not that big a fan of running!

I love various virtual race challenges on SparkPeople.com. People can come together online, yet compete and train on their own. These challenges are fantastic, and I did my first 5K race in a SparkPeople challenge! I got the chance to do it on a machine that was very much like an elliptical. Using that as a template, I have completed a triathlon by swimming in a pool, then spinning on a stationary bicycle in a gym, and then hopping on an elliptical in the gym to finish it out.

The biggest takeaway I've gotten from triathlon conditioning is cross-training. By mixing my routine up, I keep from getting bored or staying at the same fitness level. Adding in different components, exercises and various interval types of training have kept my body and my wits striving for the next level of excellence!

Challenge:

Now that you've started a team, signed up for a race (remember your assignment from Reason #56?) and are ready to start training for it, find an online challenge (or create one of your own) as part of your training. Remember – races are fun, and you don't have to run the whole thing nor compete for time. It's all about the spirit and community of it! Encourage your race team to participate in the online challenge together, and encourage one another as you train and complete the challenge.

Start training on your next workout day!

Different race organizations have helpful training guides. Here are a few:
SparkPeople virtual race guide
The Color Run
Tough Mudder
Spartan Race Workout of the Day
Beginner Triathlete

The links to these training guides can be found on my website here:
http://mindheartswole.com/swole/

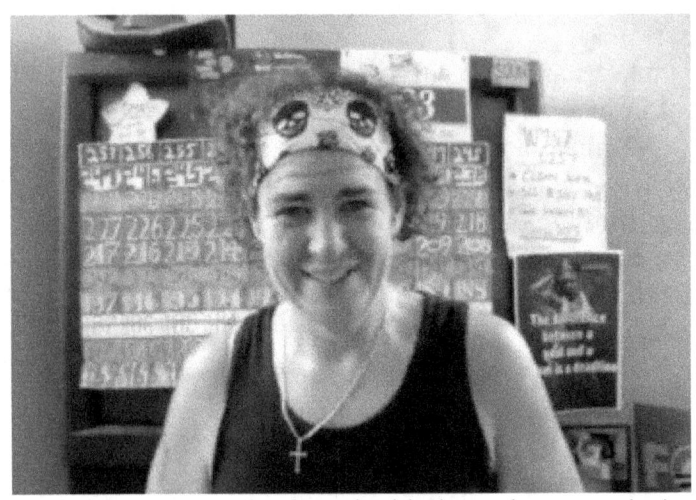

Reason #59 – <u>To get back at the bitches who try to (__) me</u>
Recorded in late August, 2013

For a while, I imagined that my success would make me feel better than (or even superior to) people that would do or say damaging things to me. I was still in the comparative, ego-based, win-lose mindset. I still had a lot of healing to do, especially when I wrote my list and started this project.

Now, I know that win-win is the best way think, act, and be. As I do well, I make it a point to congratulate people on their achievements. It's not a threat when another is successful. Cheering others on seals our own success, because if we can be proud of ourselves AND for others, we're true winners in heart and mind!

From the video for this reason:
When I wrote this list, I was having some perception issues. Perception comes from a combination of things. It comes from experiences that we've had in the past that judge and shape how we view the future, and it comes from being cynical...but also, that experience comes in.

As we wish for the best things to come into our lives, let's also pray that others get exactly what we want for ourselves. When everyone wins, there's no need to compete. Winners know this well!

Activity:
Find a container, jar or large cup that you can decorate, label, and use to place any thoughts, concerns, and feelings that trouble you. Add any harmful desires that have been pestering you, any grievances, annoyances, and things that anger you. Name this jar something positive: "Transformative Thoughts," "Released Regrets," or anything you please. Mine is called my "Stuff for God to Handle Jar." Once the jar is full, go outside and burn the notes you've added to it (I burn mine in my fire pit). Meditate and pray as the papers turn to ash, imagining that, like the paper, those thoughts and the energy is transforming into something better. Release any feelings holding you back, send them off, and burn them away.

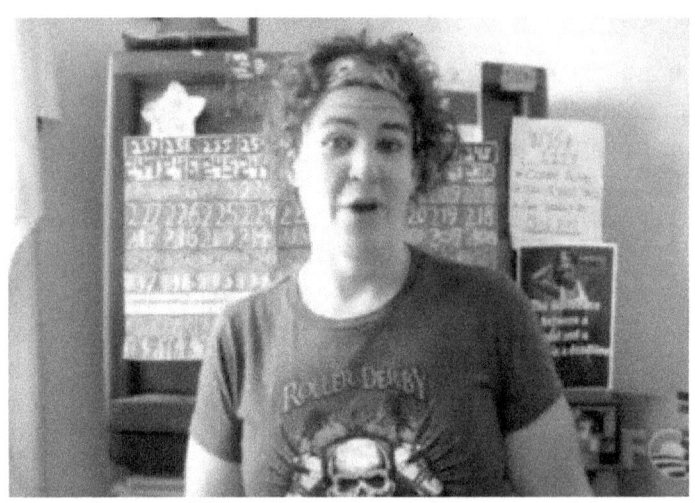

Reason #60 – <u>To hold myself accountable</u>
Recorded on August 31, 2013
Weight: 171 pounds

Accountability is a HUGE component of any lifestyle adjustment, and if we are truly to be successful, we must be aware of what we are doing, why we are doing it, and how to address problems. Accountability takes courage, and successful people are brave. It takes a lot of emotional intelligence to admit where we've fallen short, and it takes strength to take action.

A lifestyle adjustment requires better habits, and accountability is imperative to gauge what is working and what needs adjusting.

No one else can do it for us. We alone are responsible for our results. We can have people help and support us, but ultimately we are solely responsible, and wholly accountable for our wins and our setbacks.

We use blame, excuses and situations to rationalize our behaviors (especially the behaviors that keep us from our greatest good). When we take a moment to pause and own up to our actions, then we can reflect on the habits, reactions and tendencies that cause us to act that way. Upon reflection, we can then come up with action steps to get better results. Mistakes are great teachers! Learn and move on from them.

Success begins with holding ourselves accountable, having integrity, and tapping into the courage to look at ourselves honestly. When we take ownership of our actions, we can then take positive steps forward to do better.

Assignment:
Review your weekly schedule, nutrition and mood logs. If you're behind on this, take this opportunity to start right now (remember – there are 52 Mondays in a year, and 313 other days!). Keep this going for at least a week. Continue to look for patterns, setbacks and any areas that need improvement. Make sure you're planning time in your schedule for rest, meals, workouts, work, and relaxing!

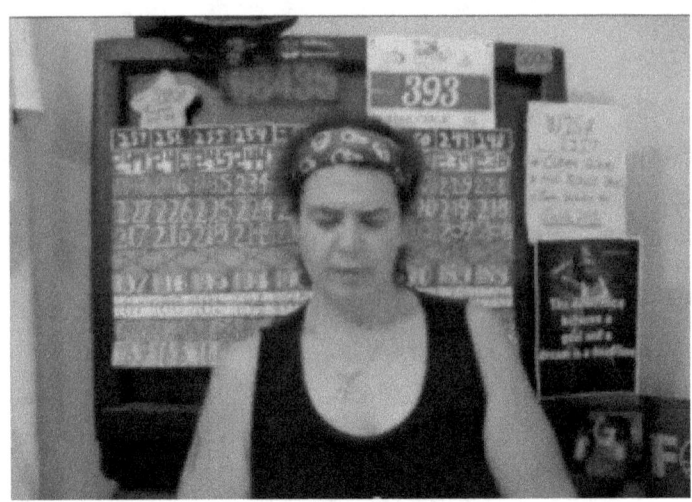

Reason #61 – <u>To be a beast in arguments</u>
Recorded on September 3, 2013

Accomplishments inspire confidence, and that empowers us to feel stronger and stand our ground whenever we face adversity. However, we can still stand firm in our beliefs while also working with others to see their perspective. Many times, we can find a balance and continue onward, even if we don't agree. Sometimes though, we must stand firm and hold true to what we feel is just.

Unfortunately, arguments can happen, and it's important to have the confidence to stand for what is right.

Being healthy creates a clear mind, and thinking happens in a much more logical, linear manner. The confidence is an added bonus, and healthy habits create healthy thinking.

Sometimes, the biggest arguments we face are the ones within our minds. By taking better care of ourselves, those racing thoughts calm down, and the reward of accomplishment quiets the busy thoughts going on in our heads.

When we accept ourselves, we have the courage to walk away from anything holding us back. We should all exercise good judgment to see which arguments we need to just walk away from (even if we're right, there are times when it's best to leave it alone), and which ones we must engage in. However it plays out, it's a best practice to remain calm, objective, take deep breaths, and speak from the heart and with logic, instead of act purely from emotion.

A wise friend of mine gave me this life-changing advice: "Choose your battles, and don't burn bridges."

Keeping this practice helps us find peace in our environments, our relationships, and most importantly, within ourselves.

Questions:
What are some things that people do (at work, at home, etc.) that make you want to argue with them?
How can you resolve a dispute without arguing?
Can you walk away from a conversation with someone you don't agree with? Why or why not?

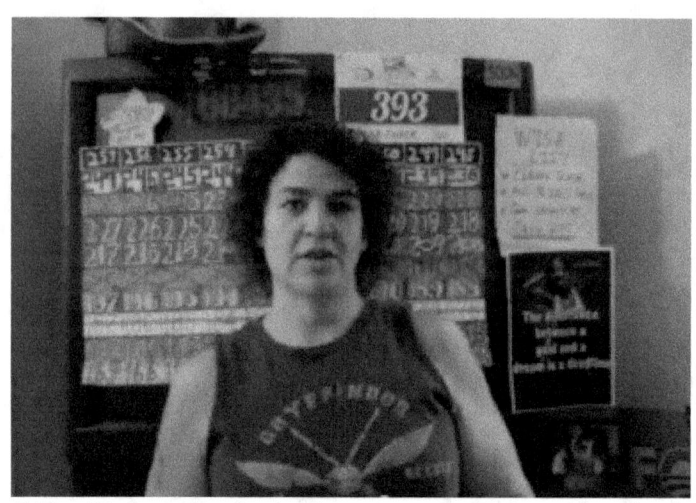

Reason #62 – <u>To be a leader in the group and not get lost in the crowd</u>
Recorded on September 4, 2013

This reason stems again from confidence, just like the last reason. In order to effectively lead people, we must believe in what we're espousing, otherwise we're full of shit, and people can see right through that.

So often, we see and hear stories about leaders who were caught in a scandal, and it's sensational because it goes against that which they stand for.

We as a people, on the whole, want to go with the flow, to get along, and to be liked and appreciated. It takes a great deal of integrity and courage to stand tall and be a leader, to inspire change, and to encourage people to go against the grain and move toward a higher ideal. So often we fall to malaise and mediocrity. We're so capable of much, much more. There's so much good in this world and it's meant to be shared; truly we can all win.

That thinking goes against the grain of common thought, but if we all realize how much we're capable of and have the strength to develop the habits to reach our highest potential (and continue to grow from there), then we learn to think in amazing, revolutionary, progressive and forward-moving ways. We see people as collaborators instead of competition. We have confidence that, even if there is competition, we'll still succeed.

Leaders are mavericks, and in order to lead and inspire people to do extraordinary things, we ourselves must be willing and ready to do extraordinary things. That requires both the strength to stick with a plan, and the humility and vulnerability to admit when we need help, support, and encouragement. No one is perfect, and we don't have to be. We just have to be ourselves, and we should be continually working toward becoming our highest selves.

These things sure sound great, right? The words can be found in leadership books, business guides and many life coaching works. The experiences, however, come from exactly that – *experience*.

I have messed up countless times, and failing is just a part of the process of growing. It has taken me my entire life to get on track with my health. There were always excuses! The world owed me a debt, all this shit had "happened to me," I would *always* find a reason to be angry, sad, to beat myself up and allow others to treat me poorly. Though I knew for a long time that my behaviors, my thinking and my habits would have to change, it just had to happen when I was ready for it. I was fed up. Change had to happen, or I was going to continue to live as a sick, anxious, medicated, using and boozing anger-monger.

As Gandhi said, "be the change you want to see in the world."

If we want to inspire people, we must be inspired. If we want to see the world healthy, we should practice good health in mind, body and spirit. Words only go so far.

Actions speak the loudest.

Lead by action, and watch in amazement how you'll empower others!

Activity:
Invite someone you admire (friend, colleague, mentor, etc.) for coffee, lunch, or dinner, and tell this person that it's on you – you're treating him or her! Thank this person for having great influence on you, and ask him or her about challenges overcome, and how he or she did it. Ask about personal stories, and listen attentively. Put away any distractions, turn your phone off, and absorb what this person is telling you. If needed, take notes (I sure do!). Learn from this person's experiences and adopt some of his or her best practices in your life. You'll be amazed how much someone is willing to share if you just ask!

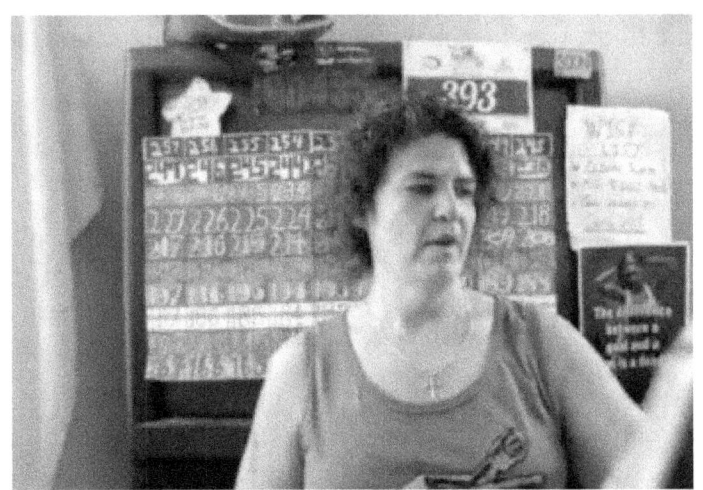

Reason #63 – <u>To be an awesome Cato</u>
Recorded on September 11, 2013

Any <u>Hunger Games</u> fans out there? Anyone? Any cosplayers out there?

Well...anyway...

Cosplay (costume play, or playing in costume as a character) was a great way to have fun, meet creative and interesting people, and just escape into a different world for some time, and pretend, just like we did when we were kids on Halloween or on dress-and-play days. It's a challenging and rewarding hobby, and while I was involved with it, I enjoyed it very much.

One of my reasons for getting in shape was to cosplay as Cato from The Hunger Games. In the movies/stories, Cato was a super athletic character who had trained his whole life to become a champion of The Hunger Games competition. The training and athletic aesthetic appealed to me, and he was the first character in a while who I wanted to portray in costume.

A friend of mine actually pulled it off quite well, and that satisfied the desire to see a great Cato cosplay. Nevertheless, this reason still inspired me to lift weights and change my body composition, so overall it turned out great! Having a visual reference gave me lots of ideas about the results I wanted, which affected how I trained. This is another example of how powerful visuals are!

Nowadays, when I close my eyes and think of my dream cosplay, I think of the same cosplay that every Star Wars fan dreams of – Princess Leia from Return of the Jedi. That bikini...yeah. I'd rock that!

Questions:
Have you ever wanted to dress in costume (for Halloween or...come on, use your imagination!)?
Have you ever wanted to get into shape for an event, like a wedding or a birthday party?
Why?

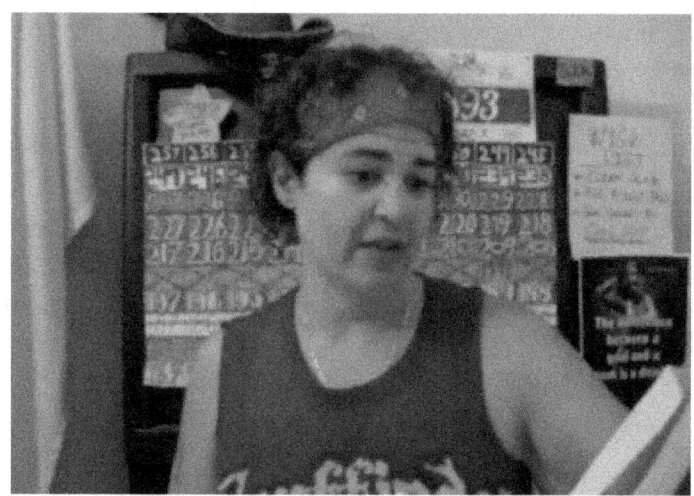

Reason #64 - <u>Despite what people say, at least I won't be fat anymore</u>
Recorded on September 12, 2013

The reason in its entirety is:
Because I've wanted to, and though people don't say it to my face, I'm still called 'fat'. I can't control what they say and it'll change if they hate me anyway, but at least I won't be fat anymore.

This one was all about internal projection, and letting my mind run wild about how people think of me and perceive me. Again, this list was written when I was 100 pounds overweight, and I was still struggling with internal and external perception issues. I wanted to be accepted for who I was, and yet I still felt like I should be judged for being overweight.

Classic human contrast; cognitive dissonance in action!

I had been overweight for most of my life, pretty much from 16 years old into my early 30s. Weight management and fitness had been very elusive, and between battling various addictions and having very little self-worth, I descended into a downward spiral in which I saw no end. That was, until I had been in various situations and relationships where I found that I was being treated poorly.

To do that to myself was one thing, to have others treat me that way was intolerable.

I thank God for those catalysts, because they woke me up and helped me realize that the only way to allow love into my life was to let it begin with me. The only way to live a healthy lifestyle was by making the commitment to follow through on it. The only way I was going to walk the path of wellness was to start taking the steps, and continue moving onward.

This is an amazing, progressive, and beautiful process in which I am always learning along the way and always finding room for growth. As long as I'm consistently seeking my greatest good, I have no regrets.

It's taken a long time for the realization to hit me (as I write this it's been over a year since I hit my goal), but I finally understand that the words and actions of others have no bearing on my personal value.

How others speak of us isn't a reflection of us, it's a reflection of them.

In the end, it doesn't matter what is said about us. What matters is how we feel about ourselves.

By taking care of ourselves, we engender love from within, and allow it to come toward us!

Assignment:
Take at least 10 minutes and write down the harshest things you've ever been told. Then, write down the three harshest things you've ever said to someone. Put these in your release thoughts jar that you made in Reason #59. Then, in your journal, write at least three of the nicest things that anyone has ever said and/or done to you. Journal about this experience.

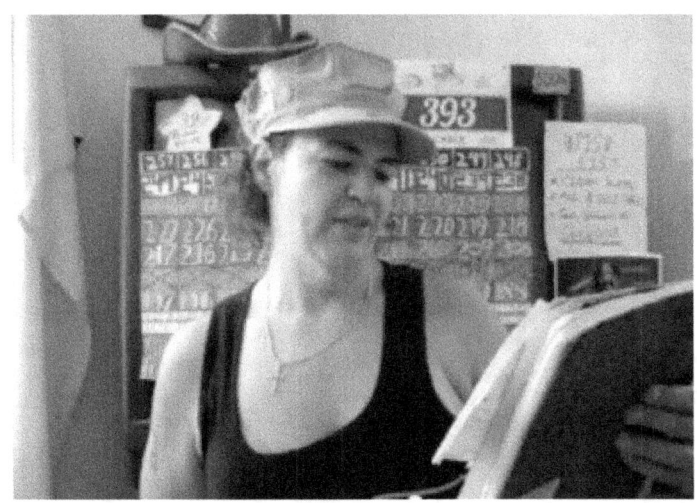

Reason #65 – <u>Because my past is in the past, and I want to leave it there</u>
Recorded on September 14, 2013
Weight: 171 pounds

Second chances are where it's at, for real. Every day, if we allow it, a clean slate is possible. We're given opportunities to try again, to find forgiveness, and to create a better life. The big trick is allowing ourselves to perceive and receive them – that can be challenging!

We judge ourselves very harshly, and this leads to all kinds of self-abuse: addiction, heart disease, staying in bad relationships, allowing an employer to treat us unfairly, choosing ego-based pleasures over the heart's desires…the list goes on and on. What we really want, what we really need is love, acceptance, and mercy. These begin within.

The past is in the past. The present moment is all that matters. With faith, hope and serenity, the future is so, so brilliantly bright.

What better way to get over the past than by seizing the day? It happens *EVERY* day. Every day presents the chance to boldly move forward, despite what happened before, despite what may come in the future.

All we have is moments. Let's make them count!

Questions:
What are some things you've been holding onto that make you feel badly?
How would you like to shed those things?
What needs to happen for you to let something go?
Does your pride ever get in the way of your progress? Why or why not?

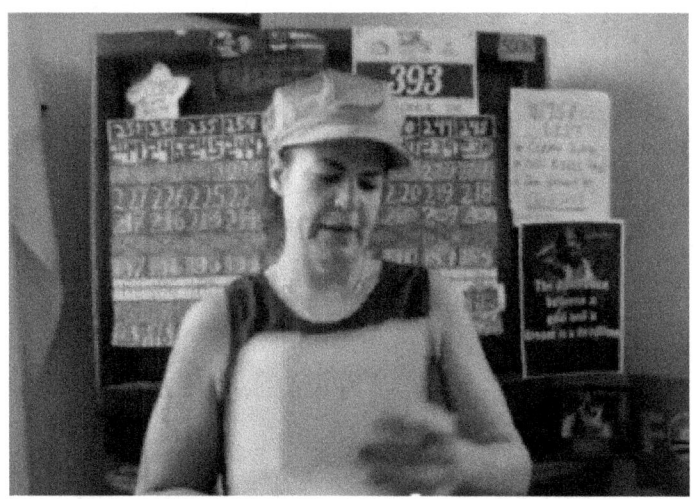

Reason #66 – <u>So people will treat me better</u>
Recorded on September 17, 2013
Weight: 168 pounds

When we feel good, it's obvious. It attracts lots of attention, and a lot of it is well-wishing, kindness, and accolades. That's all good stuff! People appreciate happy, attractive, and compelling people. They aspire to have the same, and those who can appreciate success are successful themselves.

Many of us are not born into wealthy, emotionally stable families. Many of those who do live that life earned it the hard way. It's the same with creating a healthy life. After all, a healthy lifestyle is just another success. If we don't have it, we must earn it. When we earn it, we take care of it. As we take care of it, we take much better care of other things in our lives. It's remarkable how that, in turn, affects how people treat us.

People treat us as well as we allow them to, and they only treat us as well as we treat ourselves. We can influence how others treat us (and have total control over who we allow into our lives), but we alone are wholly responsible for how we treat ourselves.

Treat yourself well. That's what matters the most. Choose your circle wisely. Just like clearing out our homes, our social circles can always use upkeep and maintenance. Sometimes we have to clear out that which no longer serves us. It may be difficult, and it will make a huge impact on your choices, habits and attitudes. If something or someone is dragging you down, evaluate if it's benefiting you. If not, it's time to let that thing or person go.

What we allow will continue, so why hang onto something that's holding us back? We deserve great things!

Assignment:
In your journal, write a list of how you think you deserve to be treated. Next, write a list of how you think your favorite person should be treated. Once you've completed that list, the final list is how you feel your least favorite person should be treated (it may be someone you know or don't know – feel free to take it out on your least favorite politician!).

After you've completed all the lists, write down why you feel each respective person should be treated that way. Then, switch it around so that the reasons and treatment take turns with each person – you, your favorite person, and your least favorite person.

Contemplate this, sit with it for a while until you can go through this assignment without having emotional attachments. Journal the experience.

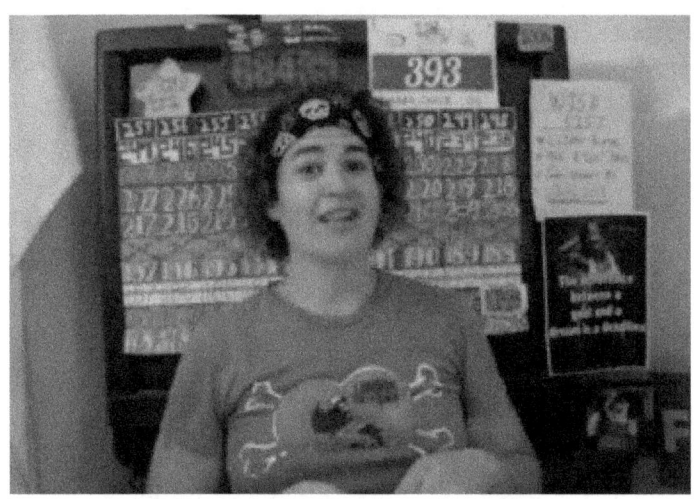

Reason #67- To get over it, and move on
Recorded on September 19, 2013

We may never truly get over something, but we do learn to live and move forward. Sometimes things come back and bite us, and we may even fall into old habits. There's always a chance to do better the next time we're faced with the same situation.

Mental wounds leave scars just like physical wounds. It takes much longer to heal from the injury than it took for it to be inflicted, and the scars stay with us. We just learn to live with them. They become part of who we are.

From the video for this reason:
The things that were going on in my life were echoing some historical things, and it is time to change how I think and how I react now to stop repeating that history. Quite often when things happen to us in life, we don't quite get over it, we just learn to live with it. Learning to live with being a 'fat girl' on the inside is going to be something that I live with every day, and I just have to learn how to manage it well. So far, things are going well.

Our experiences make us who we are. We can't control what has happened to us, we can only control how we move forward, which is completely up to us. Nothing can change the past. With tools, resources, and lots of great influences, we can learn from every experience and grow. Sometimes we have to repeat the same mistakes over and over until something *finally* sinks in. We ultimately learn that nothing changes if we keep doing the same damn thing! Doing something different is hard, and that's why we reap the lessons we've learned from each mistake.

I wrote this list when my heart felt broken. I hoped that losing weight would cure my pain, that I would be able to get over the hurt I was feeling. The end goal, to me, seemed like the solution. What I have learned is that things happen, old thoughts and feelings come back up, and it never truly goes away. The difference now is that I make better choices. I move forward; perhaps that's not moving on altogether, but it is moving in the right direction!

Activity:
Cut a sheet of paper into a heart. On the heart, write words, phrases and things that you've been carrying around that you wish you could move on from. Write anything and everything that comes to mind. Then, tear up the heart and walk away from it. Take ten deep, mindful, cleansing breaths.

Finish this first part of the assignment before reading any further.

Come back to the heart, and on backs of the torn the pieces, write feelings that you LOVE to experience. Write names of people who adore you, inspire you, and make you feel accepted, loved, and complete. Then, tape the heart back together and add it to your board/collage from Reason #5, with the positive side facing out.

In your journal, write about how this activity made you feel.

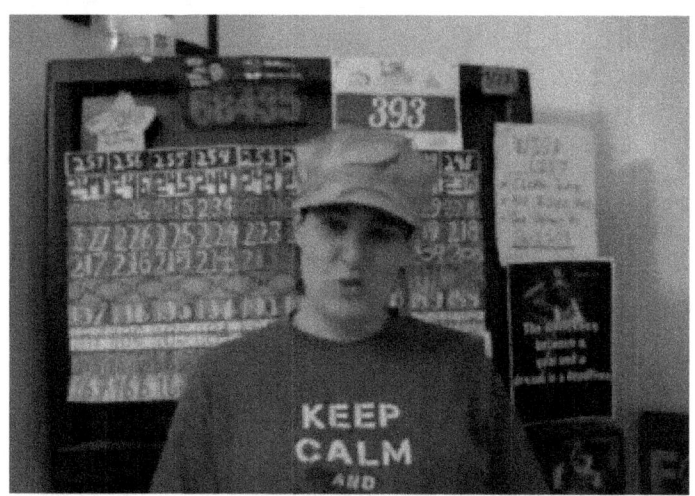

Reason #68 – <u>To attract better things into my life</u>
Recorded on September 22, 2013

We attract what we think we deserve, so let's just allow great things into our lives – we've earned it, and we deserve GOOD things!

When I wrote this list and started on this lifestyle adjustment, I wanted to leave the broken pieces of my life behind me and start with a clean slate. It's taken a lifetime to get to this point, and will take a lifetime to maintain it— the only way for me to keep a healthy lifestyle is by maintaining it every single day. This project is the result of lots of experience; I've made many mistakes before, during and after I hit my goal. Sometimes, I've had to repeat mistakes in order for it to sink in.

For example, this Reason was inspired by the end of a relationship, and I wanted to take care of myself so I would be treated better. The next relationship I got into, after I hit my goal, echoed many characteristics of the past relationship. I fell into some old bad habits. However, just like the previous one had inspired my weight loss journey, the end of last one was what got me clean and sober! Every experience has been an amazing lesson, and if I didn't learn from those mistakes, I'd just keep on screwing up the same ways!

By focusing on good habits, good thoughts, and seeking great things for ourselves, we allow ONLY good things into our lives.

Look, shit happens. That's just life. However, we can influence ourselves with positive things, to rise above the sensation of negative news, to complain less and express more gratitude, love, and affection. When we give a good vibe, we get good vibes. When we give love, we get love. When we want to feel sorry for ourselves, bad things happen.

See how this works?

Make good choices, and witness how abundance and greatness find their way to you. It starts when we stop complaining about the things that "happen" to us – often the causality of our choices – and instead make BETTER choices!

Assignment:
Set a timer for thirty seconds. Write "I BELIEVE" on the top of a blank sheet in your journal. Then, let the timer go, and for the next thirty seconds, list everything that comes to mind. As soon as something comes to mind, write it down! After the thirty seconds pass, walk away from the list, and take five deep breaths. Come back to it, read the list and write about how you feel about this thirty second manifesto. If you like what you've written, write why. If you don't like what you see, write ideas about what you feel would influence your beliefs to shift favorably.

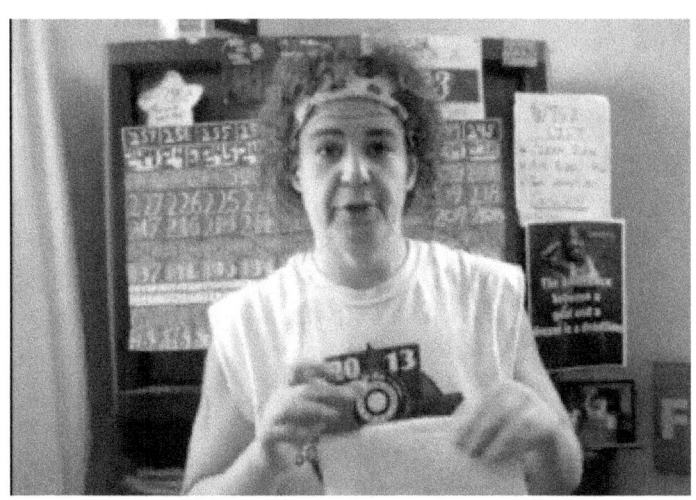

Reason #69 – <u>To understand myself more</u>
Recorded on September 26, 2013

Challenges bring our greatest selves to the surface. Without challenges, how else would we grow? We become stronger, smarter, and better by rising above adversity.

This has been a lifelong struggle for me, and the healthy habits I've cultivated and maintained along the way have shown me what I'm really made of. During the journey, the best thing I found out is that I'm totally capable of developing a healthy lifestyle and keeping it up. It's an ongoing learning process; I keep adapting, adjusting, evolving and trying new things. Every time things get difficult, I find once again I am strong, smart, and capable of surmounting anything that comes my way, and I rise to the challenge.

Someone asked me if I had always been like "this," with my defiant, can-do, driven mindset. The answer is no. It's always been difficult, and it's through uncomfortable experiences and trying hard things that I've become stronger. Every time I fall, I always get back up. Many of those times I wanted to stay down, and I sure did for a bit, but I'd get up again. Quite often, help would come my way, when I found the courage to ask for it.

The more we progress in our lives and the more we accomplish, the more we can see what we're capable of and we raise the bar.

Assignment:
Reflect on your accomplishments and moments when you've made yourself proud. Think about things you've done, how you've done them, and what more you'd like to do. You've made it this far – imagine how much further you can go! Take at least 20 minutes to journal your thoughts and feelings.

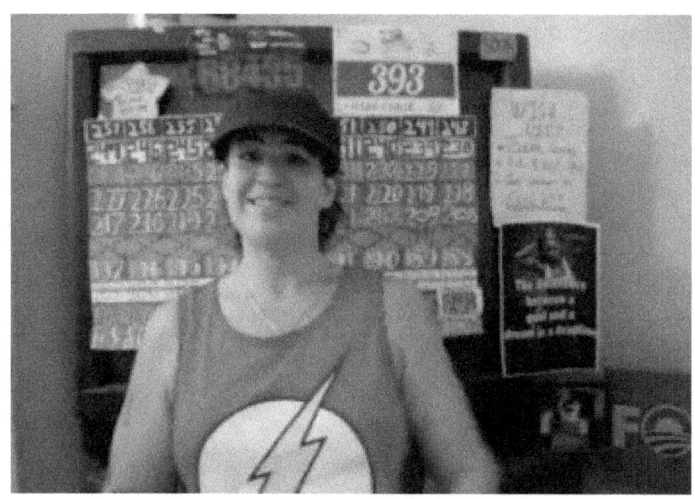

Reason #70 – <u>So my back stays healthy</u>
Recorded on October 5, 2013

Over the course of my life, I've really screwed up my back –
particularly my cervical spine! Various injuries have caused me
permanent damage, but by losing excessive fat, eating healthy, listening
to my body, practicing yoga and managing stress, I'm able to continue
to function.

Back injuries are a super tough thing to live with, and I was done with
adding more onto my hurting back by carrying around excess fat. I
knew losing the extra weight would alleviate the pain I was in and
make life much more bearable.

It's really that simple. Live a healthy life, feel better!

My back pain is drastically reduced, and I am glad to say that today,
things are going well. Granted, I do a LOT to keep myself fit and
active, and that's all part of the ongoing recovery. Even after my last
spinal injury, I was able to ease back into fitness and keep myself going
strong.

Very few things compare to the relief of recovering from a "permanent" injury!

I love shocking my doctors!

Questions:
Have you experienced physical injury? How have you recovered?
Is anything holding you back from a full recovery?
What are you willing to do to work around it?

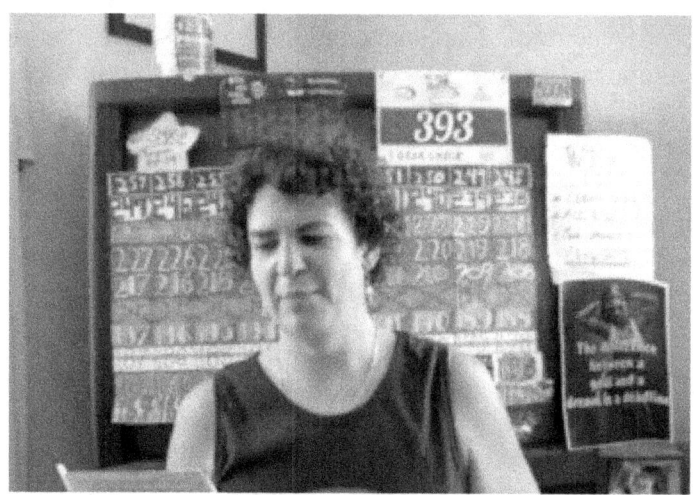

Reason #71 – <u>Because I'm happy when I'm productive</u>
Recorded on October 11, 2013

A schedule and a routine are beautiful things! People thrive when we know what we have to do, when it needs to be done, and how to get it done. A routine gives us more control of our day, instead of living in constant reactive mode. It gives us control instead of letting us *be controlled.*

We are programmed to be lazy and to find easier ways of doing things, yet we find happiness by being productive. This means we have to overcome our inherent programming and unleash our greatness by consciously doing difficult things instead of always doing what is easy.

Success begets more success. It's just like training a muscle for additional strength and endurance – the more we train ourselves intelligently (and not over-do it), the stronger we get. Surely we all have a threshold, and that threshold rises as we optimize our time efficiently.

Before getting fit, I was still VERY productive, and many of my life accomplishments happened while I was still toting around 100 extra pounds of fat. I attended a prestigious university and against many odds and hardships (including financial challenges, injuries, adjusting to a new environment, learning challenges and self-worth issues), I completed my degree with lots of work experience, and soon after secured a great job in a very competitive field and company. I defied odds and continued to be successful. For a long time, I felt like I had something to prove, that the "fat girl" wasn't lazy; she's smart, industrious, innovative, creative and resolute.

It's interesting how happy I am when I plan my day and stick to the plan. It eases the burden of having to constantly make decisions, especially where temptation is involved. For instance, when my meals are prepared and planned out, I now have more time free to focus on doing things I love. I'm happy when I get to do more things that I love!

Productivity is incredibly empowering, and the more we do, the more we can do! When we do more positive things, we have lots more to be happy about!

Assignment:
Now that you're in the habit of scheduling your week, documenting your meals and moods and maintaining a journal (even if you're not doing *all* of the assignments, you'll benefit by doing as many as you can), return again to any gaps you find. If you discover that you're not sticking to your schedule or meeting your goals, start keeping a daily activity log. Document how long you do what activities, what times, and rate the importance of each. For instance, write the time you woke up, how long it took to get ready, to make breakfast, to plan and prepare your meals for the day, how long you spent online, watching television and so on.

At the end of each day and week, evaluate your time and efforts and find any gaps. Review your goals and come up with action items to get you closer to your goals. Remember – keep it simple. Start slowly. Do one at a time. Be ambitious and yet take it easy on yourself. Work hard and work smart!

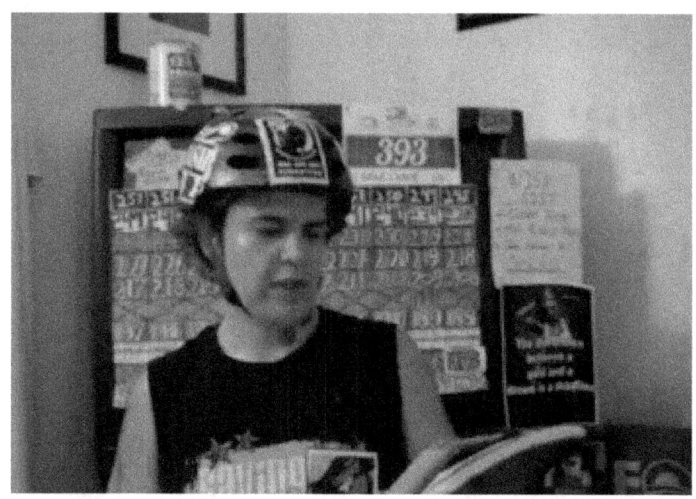

Reason #72 – <u>Because I never got myself a gift the last time</u>
Recorded on October 12, 2013

Rewards are a huge incentive to keep going! The biggest reward I've gotten myself from this experience (aside from maintaining a healthy and fit body, solid mindfulness practices and a deeper spiritual awareness) was documenting the journey. I wanted to be successful in my pursuit, and in order to keep myself accountable, I decided to chronicle the process. Recording this transition has been an amazing experience, and I'm so thankful that I've been forthright and allowed myself to be vulnerable. It's strengthened me in mind, body and spirit, and the rewards have been so incredibly amazing.

I had lost 100 pounds several years before this project, and I wished that I had documented it on film. I had a few pictures, but it was before the Facebook era, so back then, I just shared stories among friends and peers. People constantly asked me how I did it and for tips and advice, and I found I was telling many people the same thing, over and over.

That was a fantastic learning experience, and an unconscious (and probably conscious as well) part of me wanted to gain the weight back so I could go at it again, and fulfill that desire to record the transition.

So, when I gained 70 pounds back, I was given a blessing and an opportunity to carry out that wish!

It took me about 8 months to gain that weight back. That's a LOT of weight in a very short amount of time. It happened so quickly, and it's remarkable how we work so hard for something and it takes just one moment for things to fall apart. Just like any relapse, it happens in a moment, while on the other hand, it takes a lifetime to maintain the habits to stay on the other side.

What happened that caused the weight gain? I had a horrible back injury, which caused me to lose my career, leave my home, and move in with a friend until I could heal and get back on my feet. I also lost my closest family member, and subsequently fell into a deep depression. It was the first time in my life that I felt so helpless that I wanted to give up. Before this, I never imagined that I *wanted* to die, and yet during that time in my life, I was losing the will to live. My drinking was so out of control that I was using booze as a means to kill myself—I tried to drink myself to death.

Finally, something went off in my mind. I realized that humans are animals, and we have a survival instinct. How dare I go against the grain of evolution and try to off myself? So, I took a hiatus from drugs and alcohol, got counseling, worked with a doctor and took low-dose antidepressants for a few months. However, I wasn't working a program, so I was grieving, as well as drying out, without having resources and a fellowship. At that time, I wasn't ready to admit that I am an addict and alcoholic. Despite this, I stopped drinking altogether, because I knew I wanted to live (and alcohol would lead me to a grave), and I took a break from drugs. That said, addiction manifests however it can if it's not managed, and so I returned to excessive eating to cope.

A few years later, when I was ready, I implemented what I had learned from my previous experiences. Rewards were going to be an integral part of my program. I wrote a list of rewards for each 10 pounds lost and when I hit a milestone, I'd reward myself! The tattoo on right my

arm was my reward when I hit the half-way point, at 50 pounds lost.
When I hit my 100 pounds lost goal, I treated myself to my first
RollerCon in Las Vegas (in impeccable timing – I hit my goal one
week before leaving for Vegas!). I also loved spoiling myself with
clothes when I'd go down a size! The shock of getting smaller made it
hard to shop or even comprehend that I needed new clothes, so quite
often I got new clothes when I went down by *two* sizes!

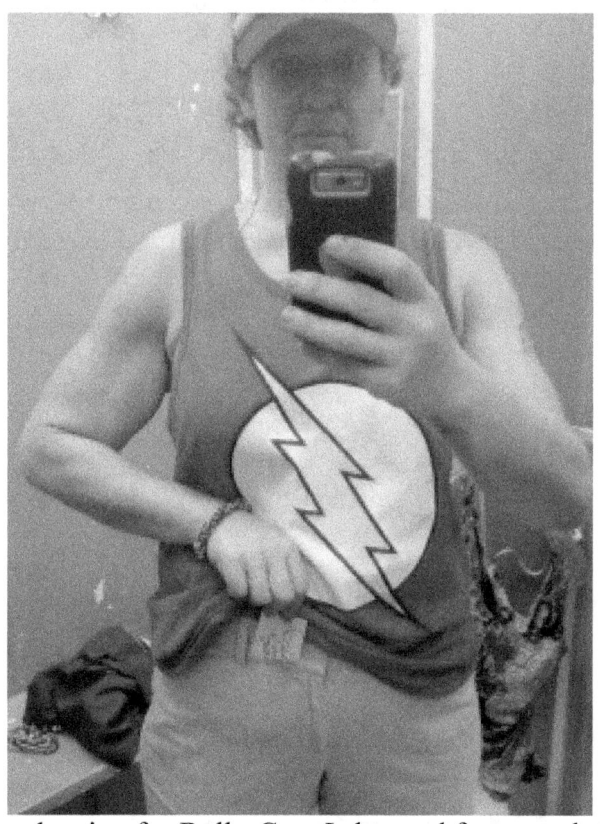

Days before leaving for RollerCon, I shopped for new clothes…and
was shocked to discover that I fit comfortably in size 8 clothes!
Genuinely SHOCKED!
ALSO! My arms!!!

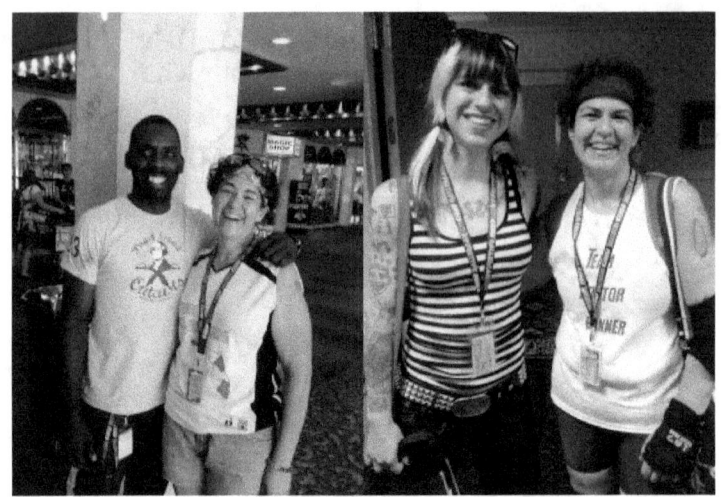

When I got to RollerCon, I met some iconic derby people! I totally fangirled when I met Quadzilla (left) and Suzy Hotrod (right), two legends in the roller skating and derby world!

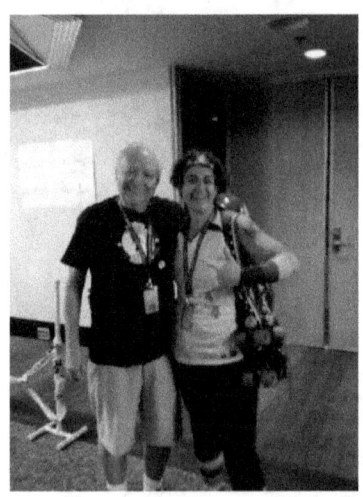

Jerry Seltzer is another roller derby icon and such a sweet man! He's a HUGE asset and advocate of the roller derby community!

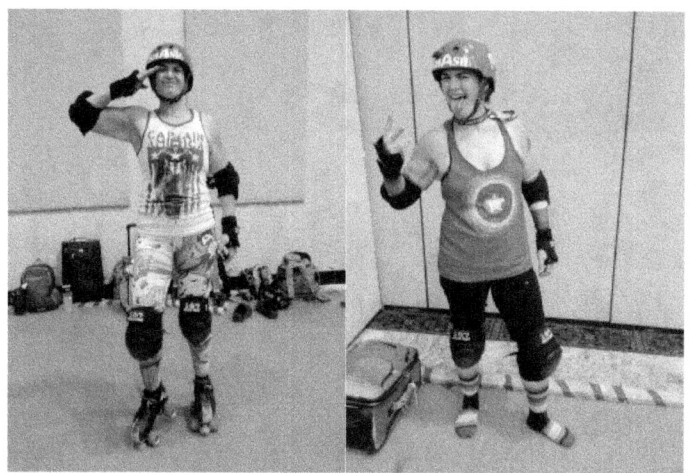

One of the best things about roller derby is that we get to dress outlandishly! I had a different boutfit for each bout...so LOTS of outlandish outfits!

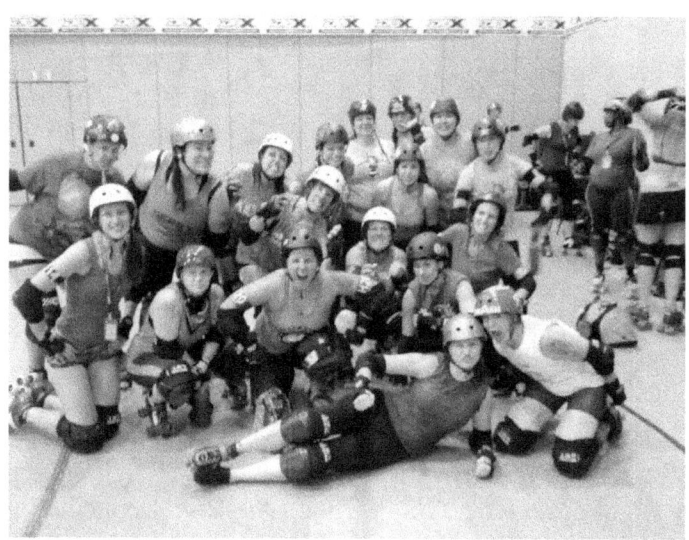

Themed scrimmages are the BEST! This was The Hulk vs. Doctor Banner!

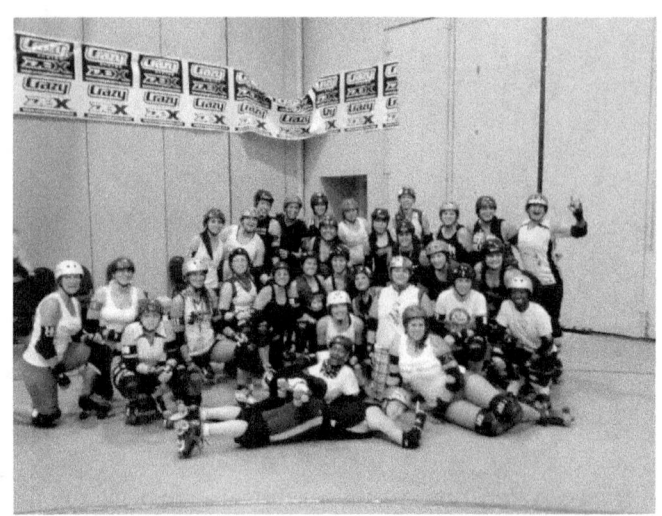

My favorite scrimmage from RollerCon 2014: North Florida vs. South Florida! It was a miracle that I got on this roster – early bouts tend to have lots of no-shows and I got SO lucky to get a spot!

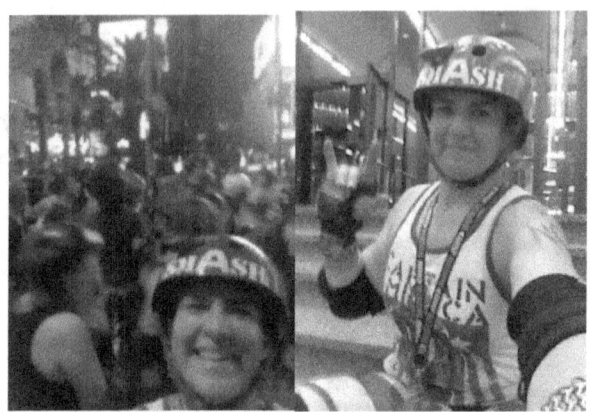

Skating the Las Vegas strip was the last event I participated in before my early flight out the next day. We left the Riviera late and got back super late. The picture on the left is me with our huge group as we set out, and the picture on the right is me just outside of the Riviera, saying goodbye. I didn't know at the time (and neither did the Riviera nor the RollerCon organizers know) that this would be the last RollerCon at the Riviera. So, my goodbye was truly a goodbye! It was a memorable and amazing experience.

Activity:

Get construction paper, colored paper or piece together several sheets of paper, and measure a strip to go along the bottom of your board that you made in Reason #5. Create reasonable milestones – 2 pounds lost, 5 pounds lost, $10 saved for a big trip and whatever else pertains to your big goal – and for each of these milestones, write down a reward voucher. When you hit that goal, redeem the voucher! Every time you give yourself a reward, photograph and document the process. See the *100 Tips for Developing a Healthy Lifestyle* for some examples, or come up with your own! Give it lots of thought! It's a great idea to make each reward progressively bigger with each huge milestone you make – for instance, make your half-way and final rewards HUGE! I went with something permanent to motivate me to stay where I am and never go back. And you know what? It worked!

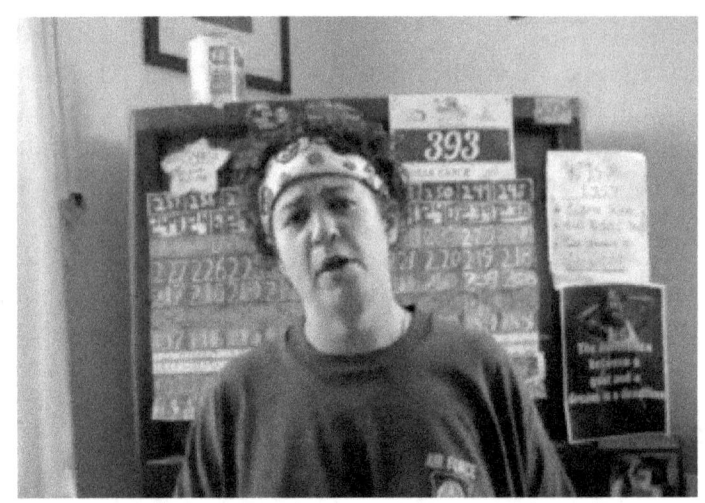

Reason #73 – <u>To take a BAMF sports bra picture</u>
Recorded Mid-October 2013
Weight: 168 pounds

BAMF – Bad. Ass. Mother. F*&%$#@! I did it!

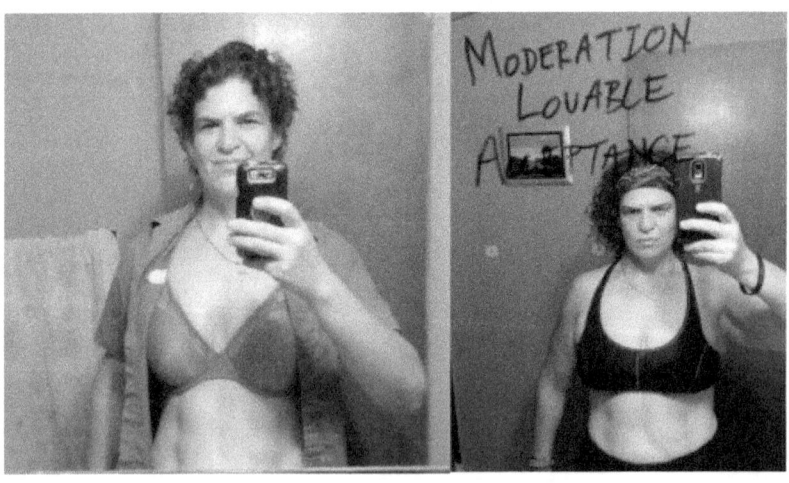

I've got a few posts on my Instagram where I'm shirtless, and there's even a video toward the end of this series where I shot it shirtless and rocking a sports bra.

There are still some body image things that I wrestle with, like pockets of fat here and there, and especially the loose skin on my belly, arms, legs and boobs. However, all those qualities are what make me unique, and it's by being unique that I'm able to stand out. I'm not like many other fitness and nutrition coaches, I'm The Dark Horse with a Bright Light (thanks to my life coach Brenda O'Donnell - http://inspiredlivingbybrenda.com/ for coming up with that one)! I'm an imperfect coach for imperfect people. My body has been through the war of a lifetime, and my stretch marks and loose skin are the scars left from battle. Yet in the end, I won! I wear my scars with pride.

Some days this is easier to accept than others, but in the long run, I've made my peace with it. I can't change the past; I can however change my perspective. I talk so much about self-love and self-acceptance, so it makes perfect sense that I have to be the very embodiment of that. Again, sometimes it's harder than other times, and that's just part of the recovery process.

Being a badass means accepting myself as I am – at my fittest, at my heaviest, at my peak, and in all the valleys in between. This goes for ALL of us.

Looking and feeling good are a by-product of this process, and it's by accepting ourselves that we give ourselves permission to work toward a goal. The work and the results are what solidify our bad-assery!

Challenge:
Write down your manifestos from Reason #68 on a loose piece of paper and put it in your pocket, and then go work out and get sweaty. No easy passes here, the objective is to challenge yourself. Working out should be challenging and uncomfortable, but not *painful*. Learn the difference. Give yourself at least 20 minutes of a good, solid workout, even if it's a fast-paced walk. Jam out to great music. Work hard for this! After you're done, take off your shirt and look at your hot, sweaty self in the mirror. Take out your manifesto and read it to yourself while looking in the mirror. Finish this off with several "I AM" empowering

statements.

Some examples are:

I AM a badass!

I AM successful!

I AM fit!

I AM worthy!

I AM free and independent!

I AM victorious!

Keep doing this until it sinks in and feels amazing! It may take a few tries, and working out beforehand will make it come more naturally – endorphin rushes are pretty cool like that!

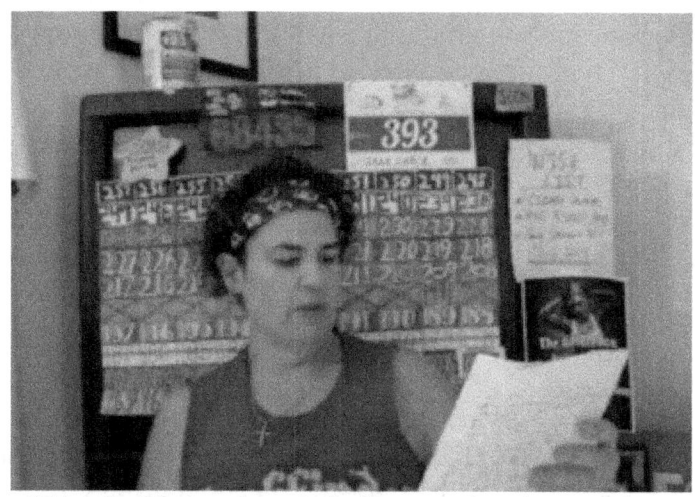

Reason #74 – <u>So I know how it feels to not be obese and overweight</u>
Recorded on October 23, 2013

Obesity had been my story for nearly 20 years, and I thought it would be my legend. I wanted to break the cycle and to create a better life for myself. I struggled my whole life to break free from that pattern.

Overeating, not exercising, active addiction and excessive drinking were all my ways of escaping from my issues instead of dealing with them. I had repressed my sexuality for 30 years, and was eating, drinking, and using drugs to escape that pain as well as numb the abuse I had experienced. I figured if I was fat, no one would want me. If no one wanted me, then they couldn't hurt me. If I hurt myself first, people wouldn't get the chance to hurt me.

Oh boy was I wrong! It made it WORSE!

I had body image issues because I was told for years that I was unwanted, that I should look, act, and dress differently. Whether I was an overly round child, an athletic pre-teen or an obese adult, I was never enough. I let the opinions of others infiltrate my thoughts and self-image. Every now and then, I'd find a sport or activity that I liked – soccer and softball when I was in grade school, martial arts when I was in middle school and weight lifting when I was in high school – but I'd gradually lose interest because the support wasn't there, because it cost too much money, and because I couldn't get a ride to and from practices. I figured it wasn't worth it if no one supported me in it. So, I then got attention because I gained a lot of weight. It wasn't positive attention, but it was still attention, and at the time, I figured something was better than nothing.

Now that I'm on the other side, I do know how it feels to not be obese and to live healthy. It feels remarkable. It's a gift that I want to share with everyone, and every person should know what it feels like to fit into clothes properly, to feel invigorated, confident, healthy, respected, admired, accepted, clean and sober. I wish I could just give it to people.

It feels fantastic to say I'm no longer obese, and I'm so thankful that I've put in the work to build this life. Feeling healthy is priceless, and if I could bottle it up and give it away, I would.

This is the next best thing that I can do – to share this journey and encourage people to come up with their own reasons and activities to fulfill their wishes and goals. It was a dream from the beginning to document this process, hit my goal, and share the journey to inspire people to get what I have!

Questions:
What was a moment in your life that you felt a huge swell of pride?
What's something you can share to encourage, uplift, and inspire others?

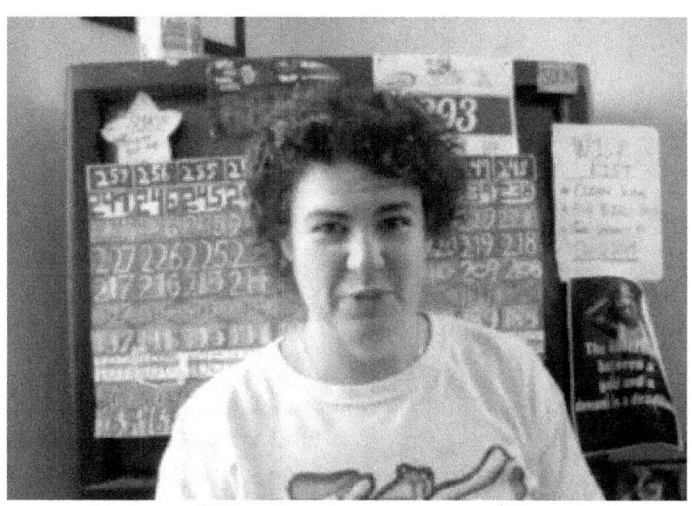

Reason #75 – <u>To piss my mom off again</u>
Recorded on November 18, 2013
Weight: 186 pounds

What inspired this reason? Look, it comes across as mean, and yes, I wrote it when I was angry. This is admittedly one I've considered editing or omitting, but I decided to leave it in. From the very beginning, I said I wanted to be forthright. This is a very human process, and anger, resentments and frustrations are all a part of it.

When I lost 100 pounds the first time, my mother asked, *"what are you going to do when you gain it all back?"* I took that comment way too personally. It's taken a lifetime to learn not to take things personally, and will be an ongoing practice.

It's great when people support us in our endeavors and successes, and when that support isn't there, it's not personal. Everyone has their own struggles.

I don't want to piss anyone off. I wrote that reason in a very unhappy and heartbreaking time in my life. I thought my success would make me feel superior to others, and that feeling superior would make me feel great.

It doesn't. There's nothing great about feeling superior over people. It makes me feel like a total flaming asshole.

There's no merit in upsetting another person intentionally. None whatsoever.

If my mother reads this, I want her to know this:
I love you. I wish you abundant health, wealth, and all the love that this world has to offer. I love you in my way, the best way that I can, from the depths of my heart with complete sincerity. May you always be blessed with abundant prosperity. You are beautiful. Thank you for giving me life and raising me. I appreciate all that you've instilled in me and I pray that you be blessed always.

Assignment:
Write a letter to someone or about something that you've been feeling a lot of anger, resentment, jealousy and negativity towards. Write it all out until every last feeling has been expressed. This may take a while. Then, take that letter and add it to your jar from Reason #59. Keep writing letters and notes as these feelings arise, and as the assignment stated in Reason #59, burn them when the jar is full. I have had to do this several times, as my jar fills up! Getting it out and letting it go keeps you from holding it in. When we hold it in, those things have nowhere to go and they hold us back. Let them go, free yourself from that stuff, and allow yourself to be rid of it. Sometimes we have to write the same thing down, or forgive someone over and over again. Forgiveness is for our benefit. Once we let that weight go, it doesn't hold us back anymore.

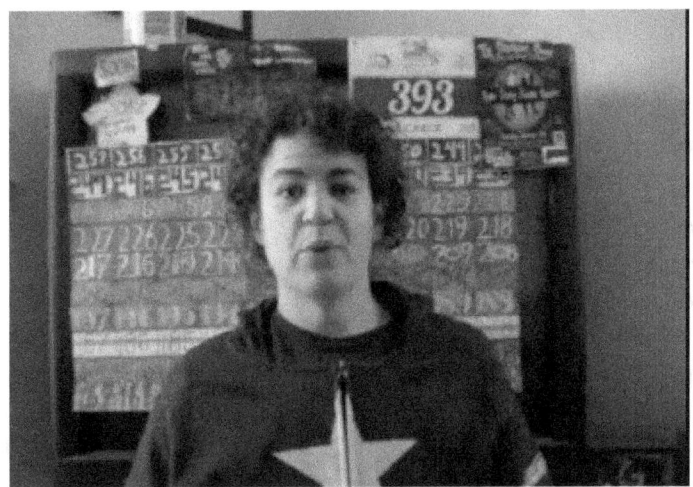

Reason #76 – <u>To get what I want</u>
Recorded on December 4, 2013
Weight: 182 pounds

When I wrote this reason, I wanted to lose all of the weight immediately. That didn't happen, but I'm glad I've had the experience to reap the insight from it. This reason is vague, and that's another thing I'm grateful for, because what I want has shifted so much from where I started to where I am now, and surely will keep evolving as I continue forward.

The beautiful thing is that life is a progressive continuum, building on from each experience. We evolve as we keep on living.

As I write this, I think about the things that I want for the people in my life, people not in my life, and our world as a whole:

- I want everyone to experience unconditional love
- I want people to be abundantly blessed in finances, health, and romance
- I wish everyone the peace and contentment that comes with self-acceptance
- I hope that luck favors all

- I pray that everyone struggling with addiction be freed from those shackles and find recovery
- I hope everyone gets a chance to read a book, enjoy a great film, and listen to the stories of people who have earned something they themselves want
- May everyone be blessed with the experience of helping and uplifting others
- May all who seek happiness find it, and keep it in their hearts and souls
- May everyone have a safe home, plenty of healthy food, and reasons to sing, dance, and laugh
- May everyone have a long-standing relationship with a Higher Power of their understanding
- May everyone experience sweeping, fulfilling, lasting romance, and that we all find someone who lights up our world and appreciates our love in equal or greater measure than we give it

And so may it be!

Activity:
Ideally, you're looking at your goals board daily, hopefully multiple times a day. The intent is to fill your mind with what's possible, and to let it come into your life. Go to your board and look it over for at least ten minutes (it may seem like a long time, so practice mindful breathing), imagining your life with these things already in it. If it needs updating, find things you want to add to it and do that after the ten minutes are up. Once we hit a goal, we should add the next. Same goes for your board!

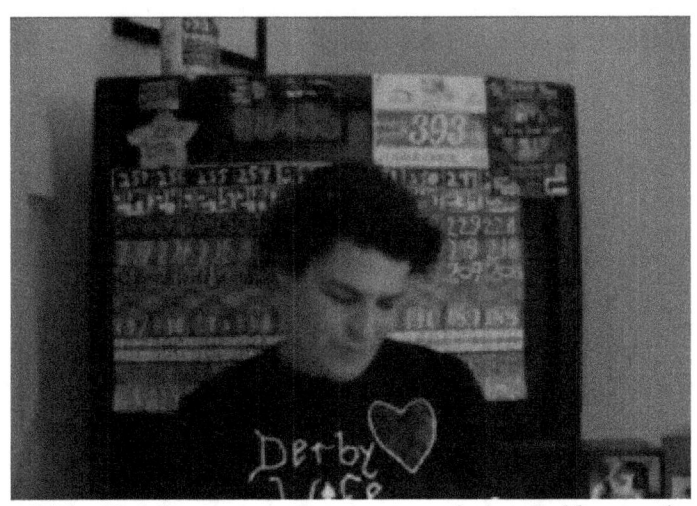

Reason #77 – <u>To show awesome progress in my self-portrait project</u>
Recorded on December 5, 2013

Just before I wrote the list of 100 Reasons to Lose 100 Pounds, I completed a photography class, and wanted to take on a self-portrait project. I thought it would be awesome to chronicle my progress in photographs as well, and I'm so grateful that in addition to documenting the process in my videos, I took some awesome pictures!

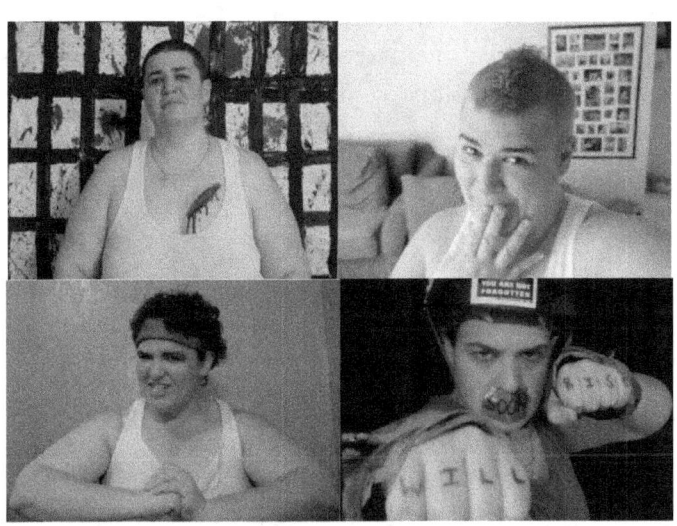

From top left to bottom right: January, March, October and then December of 2013

It worked out as well as I had hoped! When I look back at my earlier pictures and videos, I'm so proud of myself for getting started. I'm so happy for allowing myself this gift, and for finally deciding to do something about my behaviors, actions and attitudes that were limiting me. This project helped me realize that my excess body fat was a shield, a protective mechanism to keep people away. By taking care of myself, I'm allowing people to treat me better. I've been treating myself well, and that lets me allow people to treat me better.

For me, looking at the visuals puts me in a place where it's almost like my thoughts and self-perception are coming from the outside—and it's like noticing the difference between something I tell myself, and hearing someone else say it. I had tolerated those thoughts, but I'd be PISSED if someone said it to me! So, when I look at the pictures of myself, why should I allow myself to think that way? Why think and speak to myself in a harmful way?

Documenting the pictures has been great, because it helps me remember where I was, and where I am. I live it day-by-day, so seeing where I've been reminded me to keep doing what I'm doing. It's a great place to be, and I wouldn't have gotten here if I didn't get started.

Beyond getting rad pictures for their own sake, documenting and sharing my experience also kept me accountable, and to this day It also helps me see how far I've come. Every day we see ourselves, so it's hard to see the little changes. When we go back to pictures and videos from farther back, we can see BIG changes!

Assignment:
Read through your journal, especially the early parts. Look through the pictures you've been taking, ranging from your own pictures to the shots from your social gatherings. Write about how you feel now, and remember that honesty is key. Be completely unabashed in your

expression, letting any emotions flow as they need to. Happiness, anger, resentment – these are all part of the recovery process. Write, feel, and you'll work through the experience!

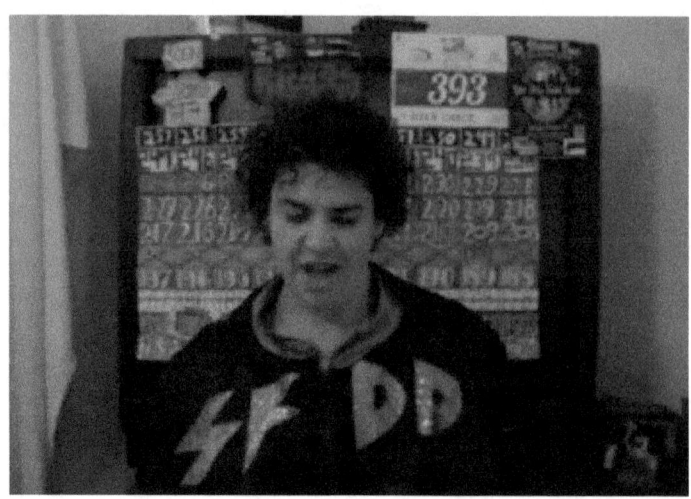

Reason #78 – <u>To get on The Chive as a hot and fit girl</u>
Recorded on December 11, 2013
Weight: 176 pounds

The Chive.com is an AWESOME website that has lots of fun pictures and memes, and I'm a HUGE fan of Cat Saturday! There is an entire section dedicated to beautiful women, and that section was definitely a big favorite for a while. My personal favorites are the women who are naturally gorgeous by being their regular everyday selves without "modeling" or trying to be cute.

As I write this, I don't feel the need to be a hot Chivette anymore. I choose now to behave the same way I'd act if I were in a serious relationship, because I truly am. I'm fully committed to wellness and keeping my head together. My sexy pictures are for me. When I'm in a relationship, I'll share them with the woman I'm with. That's about it. No more desire to seek validation as a sexy hot woman on a website. What a relief!

While I appreciate what The Chive and many other websites do for their fans and for the people who submit their pictures, it's a part of me that's in my past, and something I can reflect back on fondly. The Chive is a great organization, and they do some really cool things for their members, fans, staff, friends, service members, and charities. All the love and support for them to keep doing what they're doing – they make the world a happier place!

I'm in a place in my life where I no longer obsessively scroll through pictures of beautiful women for hours throughout my day. Admittedly, when I do see pictures of beautiful women I still have romantic thoughts, but now I let it go and move on much faster than I used to. Also, I don't feel compelled to go off into daydream and fantasy land.

Assignment:
Document your Internet time for the day as well as your nutrition, mood, work, fitness, rest, and down-time. Again, honesty and accountability are key! Look for any long stretches of time that your Internet use may get in the way of the things you need to do. Write about your needs, and take an honest inventory of the things you *want* and *like* to do, and see if they're affecting the things you *need* to do.

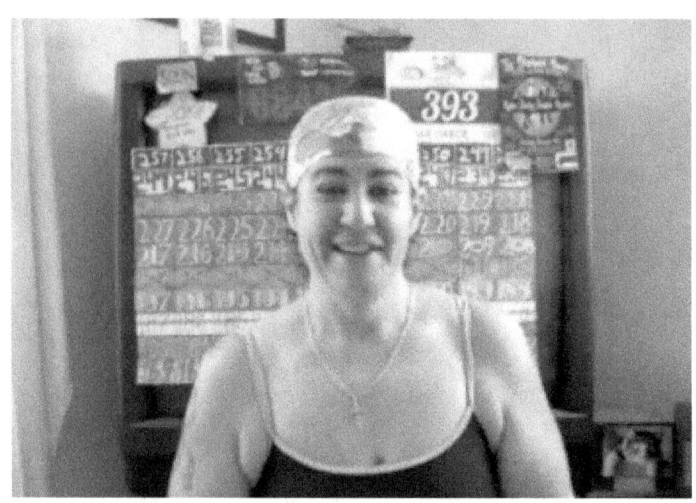
Reason #79 – <u>To get into paintball</u>
Recorded on December 23, 2013

From the video for this Reason:
There are countless reasons to lose 100 pounds, these are mine. The reasons I had when I started this list hold true now, but they are very flexible.

Paintball sounds like a hell of a great time, and I'm glad I had that fantasy for a while – it was fun to think about! Now, I know for a fact that I don't want to be shot at, and surely I don't want anything coming my way violently, even if it is for fun and sport. I've lost the taste for shooting at things, even if it's in a playful, fun environment. While I see the merit in it and fully support folks who enjoy it – have at it – it's just not something that I personally want to do anymore. I'll elaborate on this more in the next Reason.

Despite the shift in interest though, I'm still happy with this reason, because it's yet another idea I had that inspired me to get fit. I had lots of ideas about what I wanted to get into, whether they were sports I'd like to play, or ways to be active and involved in the fitness community. What I had in mind and how things turned out are completely different, and I'm thankful that I had these ideas because the pursuit has led me to find what's really good for me.

Questions:
Have you ever played paintball?
Why or why not?
Would you try archery, shooting in a gun range and target practice?
Have you done either of those? If so, what was that like for you?

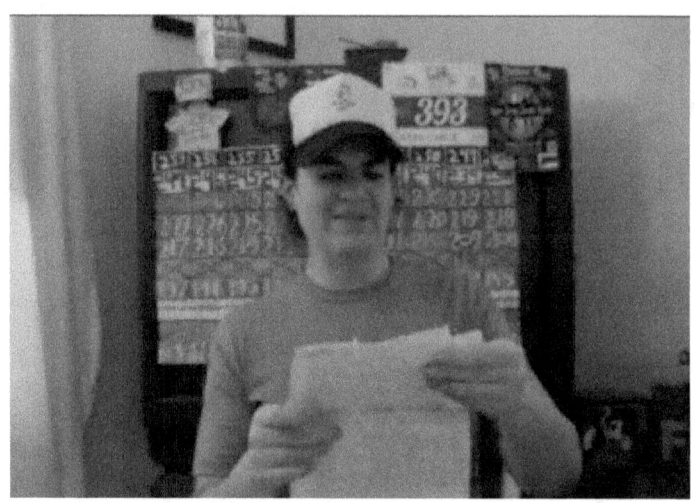

Reason #80 – <u>To be a beast at laser tag</u>
Recorded on December 24, 2013
Weight: 175 pounds

Laser tag falls into a similar category as the paintball, and while it was appealing when I wrote the list, now the appeal is pretty much gone. I tried it, and though it was fun, I've realized that I don't like being shot at or hunted (which is ironic, because I talk about hunting in a later reason)! Maybe it was the combination of everything – the dark room, the uncertainty, not being good at something right away (ugh! How frustrating!), or knowing there were people chasing me who were more experienced and skilled than I was. Being a target and at the time I tried it, I was very out of shape, so surely that was a huge turn-off!

As I write this, I realize that this experience was another one that took me out of my comfort zone. This whole experience is taking me out of my comfort zone, and that's a GREAT thing! I know now, from experience, that the things that challenge us are the things that change us. Perhaps I should give it another try. I think it's time for me to rally some friends and give laser tag another shot (see what I did there?)!

Though, I'm still not overly fond at the idea of being shot at, I have a new perspective and awareness now. Once I try laser tag again, maybe paintball will be in my future!

Since I'm holding myself accountable to this, I'll have to document it and follow up as well!

Now I'm excited to try it again! Yay for rising to a challenge!

Activity:
Host another event (or find a friend who is willing to host) and invite people over for a game night! You can play video games, board games, or anything that comes to mind! Be sure to have your guest book available for people to write in (if a friend is hosting, bring your book and pass it around for folks to write in)!

I'd LOVE to witness your experience with this! Document it – videos, pictures, social media posts – and share with me! Links to my social media and my contact information are all in this book's Afterword.

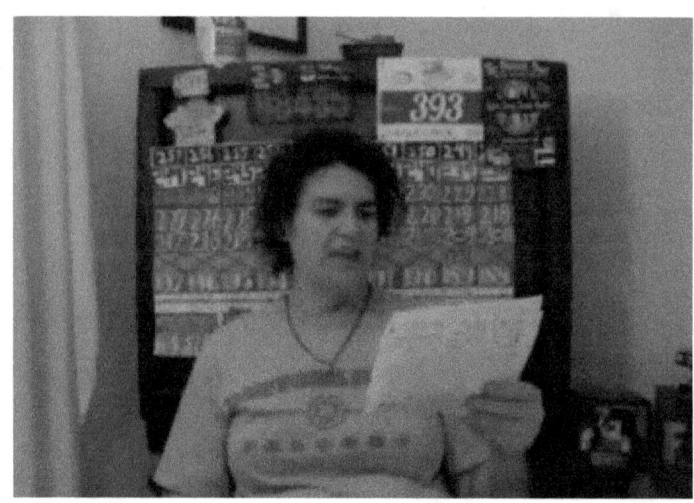

Reason #81 – <u>To catch up on all the years I've been holding myself back</u>
Recorded on December 26, 2013
Weight: 175 pounds

We get good at something by trying, by making mistakes, and by getting back up after each setback. Many of us stay in the comfort zone because we don't want to fail. In truth, failure is when we stop trying.

I held myself back because I was afraid of what my highest self was capable of, and feared the discomfort that comes with making changes for the sake of progress. I believed the lies that I was told – that I was stupid, or not good enough; that no one likes me, and I don't deserve love. Now, I know better. Success has taught me that the opposite of what I've been told is true– I'm brilliant, great, loved, and I give AND deserve great love!

It seems antithetical to go against the grain of what we've been told and what we believe. However, that's where our best experiences come from – by rising above oppression, especially when it's self-imposed (as many of our limitations are)!

The hardest part, as always, is getting started. It may seem impossible to reach our goal, yet each moment gives us an opportunity to just *try*. We don't have to conquer the world on day one, we just need to take one step forward. We make mistakes, we fall, and we get back up.

Just get started. We can't go back in time. We can make the best of the present moment. Just get started!

Assignment:
Reflect on something you've been putting off for a while. Now, do it. It can be as simple as washing the dishes, doing the laundry, or reading a book you've been staring at for months. Spend at least 20 minutes doing this activity. Just do it, right now. Then, write about your experience!

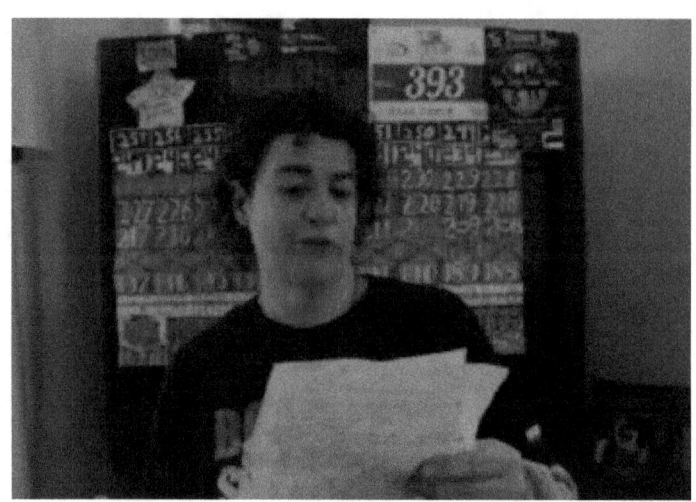

Reason #82 – <u>To striptease all hot-like</u>
Recorded on January 4, 2014

When we dress up and put on a show, the energy we feel, that surge of power and influence, comes from how we feel about ourselves. So often we rely on pleasing others to feel validated, when actually, we have the power to give that to ourselves. Only we can control how beautiful, smart, strong, capable, and successful we feel. There are many influences that can inspire these feelings, and in the end, we alone are responsible for feeling them and acting on them.

We don't have to be thin, fit, or "pretty" to be beautiful. We should just embrace ourselves as we are, in all our glory, flaws and all. Confidence and total self-acceptance makes us hot.

Gyrating hips and a pair of nipple tassels sure help, but they're not necessary. What is necessary is the presence – a smirk, a coy glance, a flirty wink, the slow removal of a glove, a shoe, the always-leave-them-wanting-more that does the trick. The only way to leave that insatiable desire is to not give it all away.

There's so much power in that!

Questions:
What is one of the sexiest things you've ever seen?
How do you like being seduced?
What arouses you?
Have you ever done or received a strip-tease? If so, what was that like for you? If not, do you want to? Why or why not?

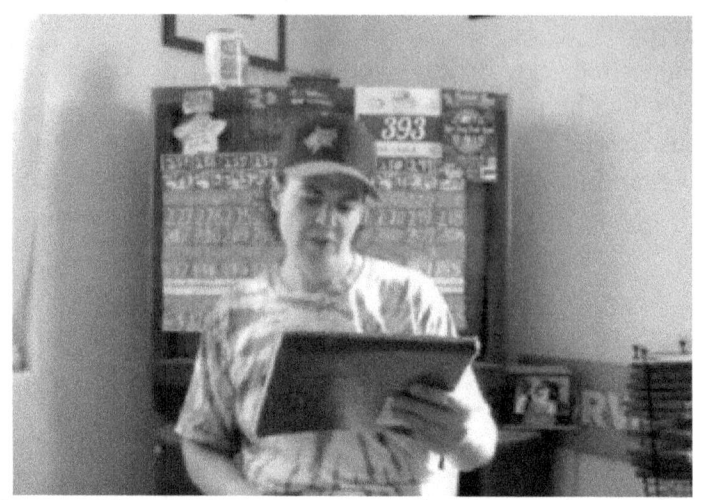

Reason #83 – <u>It'd be awesome to do a boot camp workout</u>
Recorded on January 26, 2014

High intensity intervals, boot camps, and Tabata workouts are great for building strength and endurance, and I'm definitely a witness to the effectiveness of mixing it up with training!

This reason was inspired by obstacle course races, such as Spartan Race, Tough Mudder, and the zombie 5K I did, Run For Your Lives (SO much fun!!). The training seemed hardcore, and rightly so – those races live up to their names! I was turned onto the idea of training for these races because they looked like so much fun, and because of all the great stories I'd hear in the racing communities!

What I absolutely love about these race organizations is that they provide training guides! Spartan Race has wonderful Workout of the Day (WOD) emails and a handy website, and the Tough Mudder's website has a detailed training guide. Links for these have been provided in Reason #58.

These workouts are intense and can be *very* intimidating. Frankly, if I didn't teach the classes, I would be hard-pressed to attend them as often as I do! However, we go at our own personal pace and build on from there. Students of every shape and fitness level come to these classes.

People may say they're "too hard", and sometimes I get a lot of students that try it once and never come back. The ones that succeed listen to their bodies instead of feeling compelled to follow along with everyone else.

When we listen to our bodies and hearts, we know where to grow. We know when to push ourselves, and when to back off. That's how we grow – accept where we are, intend to keep at it, and never get comfortable! There's no comfort zone, only growth!

Challenge:
Check out various workout of the day options – Tough Mudder training guides, Spartan Race Workout of the Day, the fitness app WOD Box, or anything you can find online (Pinterest has some GREAT stuff!) -- and make one your workout for the day. Go into it with willingness – remember, you *get* to do this. You *can* do this. Go at your own pace, breathe through the challenge, and enjoy the benefits! After you've completed the workout, write about this experience.

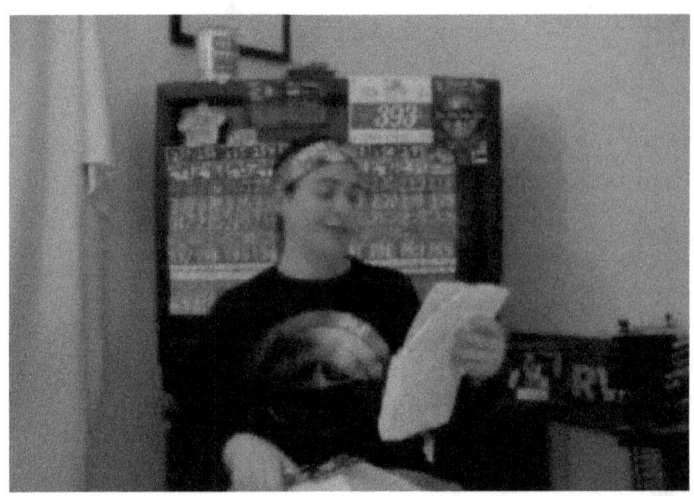

Reason #84 – <u>Because this place needs more hot lesbians</u>
Recorded on January 31, 2014

Coming out took me a LONG time. It took me 30 years to finally admit to myself and others that I'm gay. I wrestled with my sexuality for my entire life, and just like my addictions, I really thought I could out-smart it or get rid of it. It doesn't work that way. So, instead of get rid of it, I'm just letting it shine!

We cannot change what we are and how we're made. We can change our lives and make the best of it, but we can't change who we *are*. I'm so grateful to be alive in this day in age where I can openly discuss being gay. It has caused me some trouble from time to time, but that trouble is nothing compared to how hard it was to hold myself back.

I come across MANY gays in recovery. In sharing my experience and speaking with others, I find many common threads – we've been rejected, discriminated, abandoned and abused (in EVERY way – mentally, physically, sexually, spiritually, and emotionally). We have found help and hope within recovery groups (there's an LGBT group that I LOVE attending!) by spending time with others who know our struggles and have overcome them, and by allowing ourselves to be success stories, to be victors, instead of succumbing to victimization.

We take positive action instead of continue to decline on a downward spiral.

I've had some personal experiences with discrimination, and while I can't change how people act, what they say and how they think (no matter how wrong or hateful it may be), I have complete control over how I react.

I was working for an establishment that did not have gay, lesbian, bisexual and transgender protection in the equity statement and anti-discrimination policy. Working with the various professional constituency groups (employee advocates), the Gay-Straight Alliance, our Office of Equity and Inclusion and the institution's president, we ultimately got LGBT protection. Shortly after this happened, there was a rash of anti-gay comments made in various professional settings – to me, personally, in my office, and openly in a staff meeting with leadership present. In the past, I let this stuff go.

Why did I do this? I was afraid of losing my job. When I experienced a lot of name-calling when my ankle was broken, I went to my boss at the time and was told that I needed to fix my attitude. Though I do take responsibility for my reactions and my attitudes, I realized later (especially after the anti-gay discriminatory comment was made in a staff meeting) that we had a culture and organizational issue.

I went to Human Resources and the Office of Equity and Inclusion. I was still afraid, and rightly so. Ultimately, the person who was making the comments was moved into another office. Then, the organization decided to end my contract, and they gave this person my job and my office. I never asked for a reason why they decided to end my contract and I never needed to ask. It was clear, especially since they asked me not to go to the media after this ordeal.

It's taken me a while to write this out. I wrote it, deleted it, and decided to put it back in. Frankly, I don't want to come across as a "victim" and the reality is that it's been an immense blessing. Why was I afraid of losing a job in a hostile environment? I deserve way more than that! I was a dedicated, loyal, productive employee. While my attitude was an issue (I own up to that. The environment was sucking my life force like a Dementor sucks souls in *Harry Potter*), I was doing the best I could at the time.

Many people have asked why I didn't sue their asses off. I thought about it and had spoken with several attorneys about it. Ultimately, I decided to stop holding onto that anger and pain, and to do something positive with it. I spoke with the state of Florida about it and they turned my situation into a case study, so they can use my experience to educate employers. That ultimately protects people.

I'm also sharing this with you, and I hope this experience empowers you to both stand up for what's right and to take ownership of your reactions. We can't change the world around us by force, but we can inspire people by taking positive action. I was able to leave that environment and focus on my goals and dreams. It's been an amazing blessing, as any hardship can be.

Discrimination and abuse still happens, even in this age. Thankfully, there is more justice when it does happen, and more protection to prevent it from happening. People are getting more educated, and with more education comes awareness and acceptance.

There are plenty of good-looking lesbians. What this place REALLY needs is more authentic, brave, fearless, vocal, fair-minded, honorable, peace-seeking, intelligent and maverick members of the gay community who are beacons for our family, and can effectively, and respectfully, work toward maintaining a positive image, while rising above labels, bullying and discrimination.

We owe it to ourselves to be proud of who we are, to OWN It, to honor ourselves and accept ourselves wholly and completely as we are. Anything less diminishes our light, and we are made to SHINE!

Questions:
Is there something you've been holding back about yourself because you're scared or embarrassed?
What are you ashamed of?

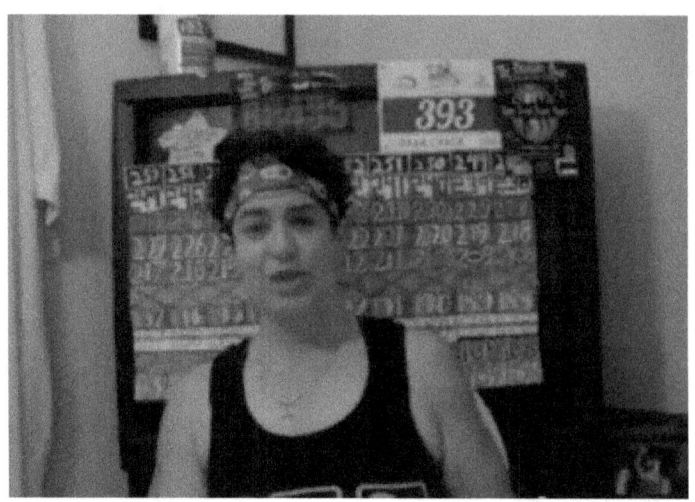

Reason #85 - <u>To take a greasy-ass bodybuilder pic</u>
Recorded on March 25, 2014
Weight: 164 pounds

Several of the reasons have pertained to photography and photoshoots, and I had a fantasy in my mind of a classic bodybuilder-style picture of myself hanging by my doorway (just like Samantha from *Sex and the City* after her boudoir photoshoot! Except hers is sensual and feminine, and mine would be all about muscle and tone), where I'm cut as a diamond, greased up, and posing all fit and toned like a true athlete and bodybuilder.

I have a lot of appreciation for athletes, lifters, and people with amazing physiques. They look amazing! I may never have that look because of the scars and loose skin that I carry around, and that's okay. I have my fitness, my health, and the feelings of accomplishment for earning this gift. I've earned that, and that is amazing!

Plus I've got so many roller skating pictures, who knows if there's even room for bodybuilder shots? I'm a bit biased here, but I think the skating shots are TOTALLY badass!

Assignment:
Find a local athlete that you admire – one of your fitness instructors, a friend, someone in your race group, a gym owner or member, a local sports person, someone you see at the gym – and speak with him or her about their training plan. Ask detailed questions about his or her fitness routine. Ask how he or she views and overcomes challenges. Ask what inspires him or her to stay on track!

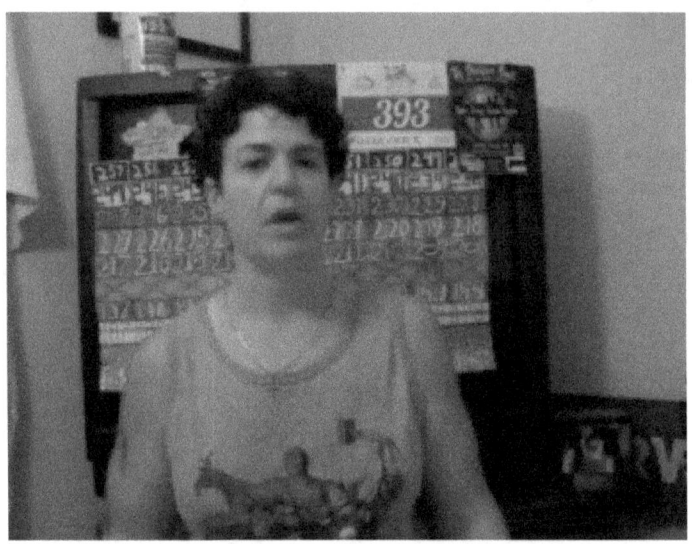

Reason #86 – <u>To take laughable clown-sized pictures</u>
Recorded on March 26, 2014

Big pants, smaller body, yay! I thought it would be fun to take some pictures in my old clothes, and one day while putting laundry away, I found an old pair of size 24 pants that used to be pretty tight on me!

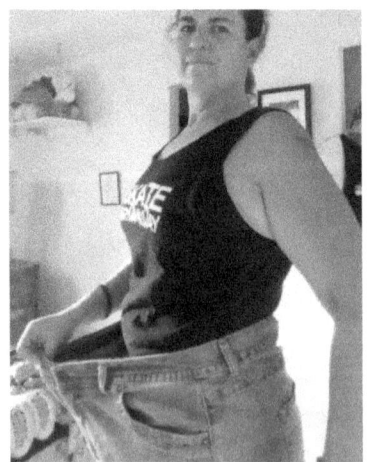

Not so tight anymore!

When I put those old pants on, a huge sense of pride and accomplishment washed over me. Sure, I enjoy the many benefits of being fit, but I still have similar thoughts that I had when I was much heavier. I know I look a lot different, and I sure feel how differently my body works. Putting those pants on really let it sink in that I've come SO far and I've got so much to be proud of.

It was a huge reward to put those pants on, and when I wrote the list, I thought it would be a humorous experience. There sure was a huge smile, but it wasn't because I thought it was funny.

The smile came from pride, accomplishment, and love for myself and the accomplishments I make each day to preserve this life, this body, and these habits that have kept me happy, healthy, and as sane as I can be!

There are moments I wish I could go back in time and give the 100 pounds-heavier Karen some words of encouragement. I'd tell her that she'll do it, tell her that she's worth it, tell her to keep believing in herself and to love herself. It all happened as it needed to, when it needed to, exactly how it needed to. It happened when I was ready, and now that it finally has, I want to keep spreading the love and sharing the message of hope to people who want what I now have. I've read in Recovery that the best way to keep something is by giving it away, and I want to keep giving people the message of self-love, self-worth, and self-care.

It happens. It happened for me, and it can and will happen for you. It's so hard to make that mental connection, to decide that now is the time. Once that realization is made, miracles happen. There are wins and there are setbacks, and there are always opportunities to get up and keep going at it.

Get started, keep going, and believe it *can* be done – and then it will happen!

Activity:
Find a "before" outfit, if you still have it. If not, go try on clothes in your "before" size. Take lots of pictures. If you're still starting out – and that's totally okay! -- put your clothes on and take your before pictures now. If you've been working toward your goals and have made some progress, take pictures now in your "before" clothes. Write about your experience, and be sure to share your pictures – it will keep you accountable, and will make you proud when you visibly see how much progress you're making!

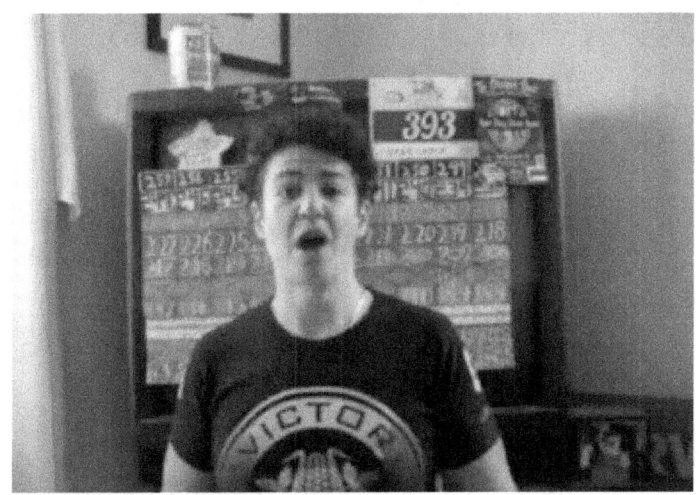

Reason #87 – <u>To shop in more stores</u>
Recorded on March 27, 2014

Shopping wasn't fun 100 pounds ago. The selection, quality and styles of clothing available just didn't appeal to me. Part of that is based on perspective – I didn't see myself looking good in what was available because I just didn't *feel* good.

Since transitioning into sizes below plus-sized, I've enjoyed shopping a lot more. I feel more comfortable, cuter and sexier in my clothes, and now I have a much wider variety of stores and styles (that I like) to choose from.

Granted, shopping still isn't an altogether thrilling process (often I ask my friends for help), and that's okay. It doesn't have to be. This process hasn't totally changed who I am; at the core, I'm still a tomboy, and I'd much rather be shopping for groceries, books, and sports equipment than clothes. Thank goodness I have friends who are more than happy to help me shop!

Before this project, every time I'd go to the dressing room, it meant having to face the reality that I had gone up in my sizes. I'd try squeezing into clothes that were too tight, trying to convince myself that I was a size smaller than I actually was. I was also putting on clothes that were way too big, thinking if it was baggy, it was comfortable and would hide my fat. Both looks were quite unflattering! Plus, I'd leave the store with clothes that were too small (in denial about my real size, and convincing myself that I'd eventually fit into that smaller size), or I'd leave with nothing at all. This behavior defeated the whole purpose of going to the store in the first place!

Gaining weight sucks. Going up several sizes (especially when it happens so rapidly) *really* sucks. Wearing the right size clothing is a step in the right direction, and allowing ourselves to just *be* that size and not change it immediately helps us take steps in the direction we want to go in. We have to work for it, and often the hardest work is first just accepting where we *are* before chasing who and where we want to *be*.

The dressing rooms are now a much more welcoming place for me. I wear what fits, without regard to the number on the label of the clothes. I've finally accepted where I am.

Doing the work and getting the results is a hell of a lot better than the suckage of wearing the wrong size, feeling miserable in clothes, and dressing sloppily!

Assignment:
It's time to window-shop! The assignment for Reason #19 was to buy a smaller outfit, and now we're taking it to the next level and going into more stores! Bring a camera (or use your phone's camera), and go find outfits that you love. Bring friends if shopping is a challenge for you (I need my girlfriends for this!). Find styles that appeal to you – not what you *should* wear, but what you'd *like* to wear. Personally, I like a mix of sleeveless tops and slacks, a few shirts with ties, and suits. Wear what makes you feel good, and makes you feel like you look good. This may change over time, so feel free to check out thrift stores!

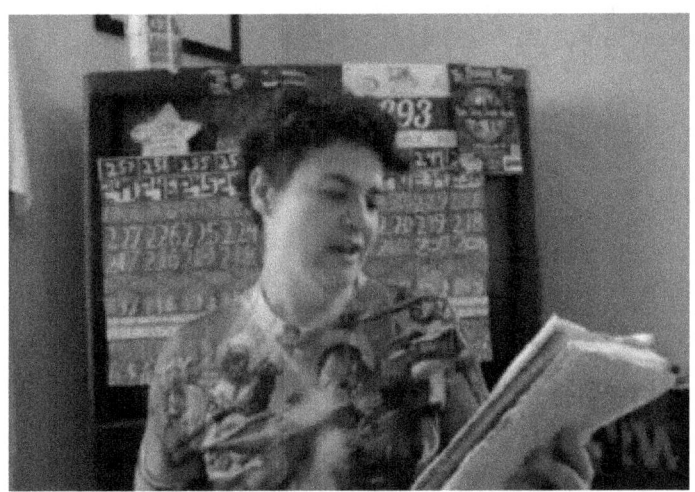

Reason #88 – <u>To finally get out of the plus section</u>
Recorded on March 29, 2014

There's nothing wrong with being plus-sized; hell I was in the plus section from the age of 14 onward. I am a supporter of <u>Health at Every Size.</u> We are allowed to accept ourselves at any size and admire the quality of person that we are. People of every shape and size are beautiful! Women of every body type are gorgeous– it's all about how we rock what we have! I've been so blessed to know, befriend, and share intimacy with women of many sizes and shapes. Beauty is more than just one image of how one "should" look. Beauty is all about how we proudly own what we have, and I sure love a woman who can confidently and proudly be her unique and authentic self in all her glory! A woman's mind, to me, is her most appealing feature. When a woman can confidently and honestly accept herself as she is, that to me is the very quintessence of beauty and it is very, very attractive!

This reason was written as a fantasy – I hadn't ever been under a size 14 in my entire adult life. When I started wearing size 12 clothing, I found more options. At size 10, there were even more. When I fit into a size 8, I marveled, shocked, at the selection of cute, fun, sexy, sporty and professional attire. I love that this reason comes toward the end, because it actually applies! I HAVE finally gotten out of the plus section! What I initially had written as a fantasy became reality, and it's extraordinary! Plus, I find a more favorable selection of clothing, in terms style and variety, and what makes me feel beautiful and confident.

Though I'm excited that I met my goal, I think it's important here to give a reminder that we are beautiful at any size, and the sizes on our clothing labels do not label us. Those labels do not dictate our state of health, wellness or level of happiness. Our size does not define who we are, how great we are, or our value.

Questions:
What do you consider to be a healthy size for your body frame and type?
How did you come up with this estimate?
Have you ever been that size?
What motivates you to fit into that size?

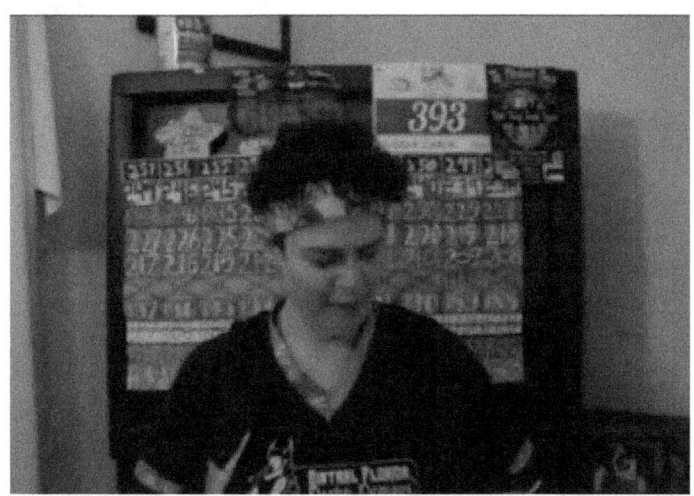

Reason #89 – <u>So I'll survive the zombie apocalypse</u>
Recorded on March 29, 2014

Everyone knows the first rule of zombie survival is cardio! So, getting in really good shape helps keep us alive!

Zombies hate fast food!

Well, whatever it is I may be running from – bad guys, real or fictional (or who knows, maybe zombies ARE real), or even the ongoing mess in my head— it helps to be in great shape so I can thunder my way through it!

Quite often when I'm working out by myself, there's a lot going on in my head. As I'm going through the motions of the workout, I imagine overcoming every challenge that I'm facing, even if it's as small as getting through the next stride or repetition. Whatever it is I'm doing, I strive to get through to the next one, breathe, and move onto the next. When it gets hard (especially in the beginning), I pray, breathe, focus on the next stride, trust my body, and keep going until I hit my goal or surpass it.

Like a lion chases the next meal, we can chase our healthy lifestyle and successfully capture it. We can also be the gazelle, running away from the bad things chasing us, trying to hold us down and away from being healthy in a pretty definitive, permanent way.

Whatever the reason for my running (or cycling, skating, swimming, lifting and so on), I'm doing it to be stronger, to survive, to thrive and rise to the next challenge. There will ALWAYS be a next challenge, and I want to be strong and fit for it.

Plus I like my brains; the zombies aren't allowed to have them!

Questions:
Are you running or escaping from anything? What is it?
How do you feel when you slow down for a moment?
Do you give yourself a break? Why or why not?

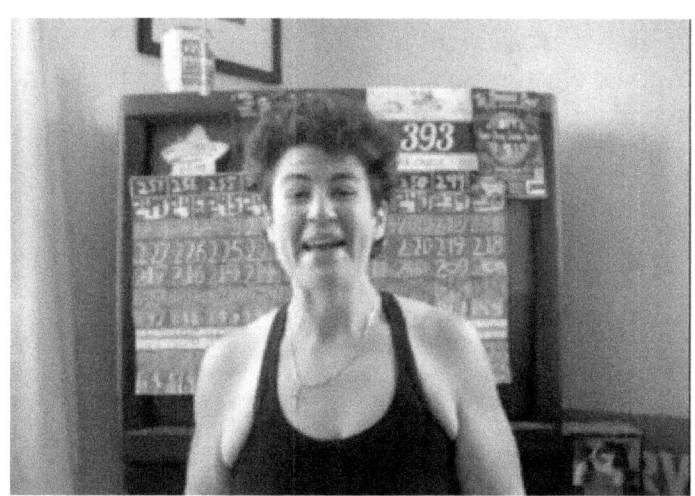
Reason #90 –To make Manda proud
Recorded on March 30, 2014

My friend, Manda, is the first person to show me true, unconditional love in friendship, and I'm so fortunate and thankful to have her in my life! We've been through a LOT together – happy and difficult times (especially when I would drink...and the cops would show up...she forgave me and I'm so thankful)– and she's been a shining light of hope, grace and inspiration for how to live with and through all the challenges that life gives us.

There have been many times where I have tried to get healthy in my life, and she has supported me in every effort. This time, I wanted to make it a point to follow through on this, to be healthy, get my life in order, and finally give her the reward for putting such faith, trust, and support in me.

The last time I saw her, I got to show her how far I've really come, and she FLIPPED out! That was one of the biggest rewards in this process. Making a loved and dear friend proud has given me the fuel to just keep taking good care of myself, to let people know that the support given to me hasn't gone to waste.

This is one of the few Reasons that's actually about someone, and I couldn't think of a better person to dedicate a Reason to. Manda is an amazing friend, and making her proud has been one of my life's dreams come to reality!

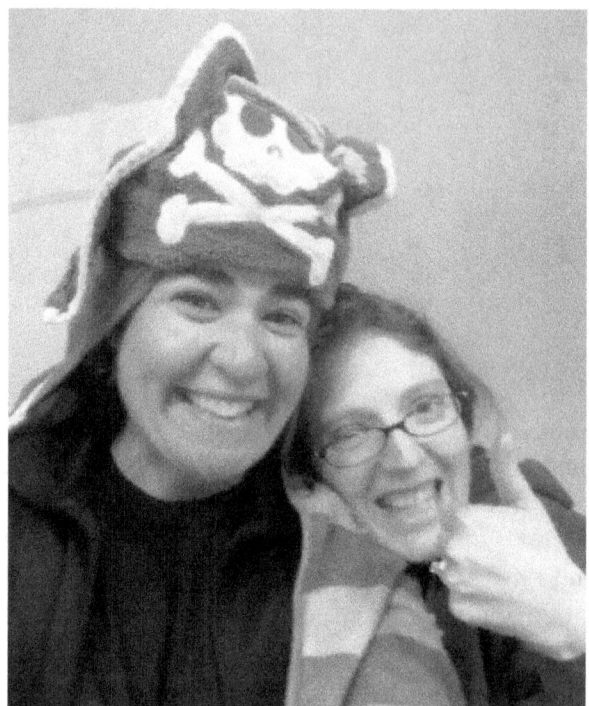

I just love her to pieces!

Activity:
Think of a friend and/or loved one that has supported you in the good times and especially the really bad ones. Find pictures of you together, get them printed and create a collage. Frame the collage, write a thank-you note or card, and give it to this person. Then, journal about how this felt, and what else you want to do to make yourself and this person proud!

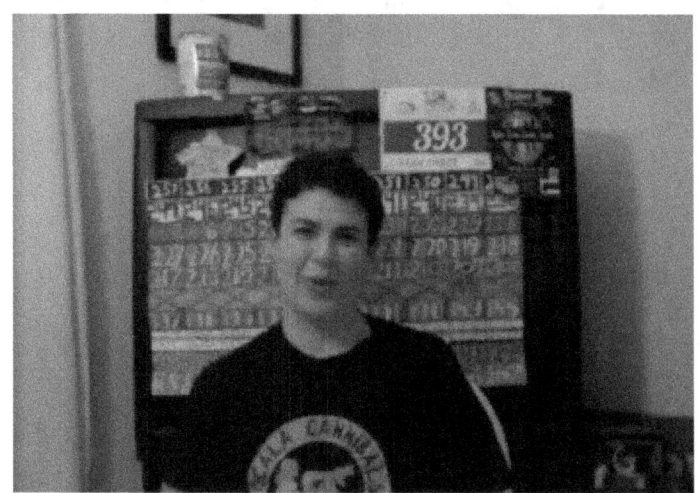

Reason #91 – <u>To outpace somebody under 76 years old in a 4-mile race</u>
Recorded on March 31, 2014

Whenever I'd run races, I found it helpful to have a pacer, someone who was running about the same speed I was and maintaining a consistent pace. While running a four-mile charity race (to raise funds for Camp Boggy Creek, and excellent organization that benefits children with serious illnesses) in New Smyrna Beach, FL, I found someone who was at my pace. I stayed right behind her, maintaining a bit of distance and keeping my pace until I sprinted to the finish line about 100 yards from the end. After the race was over, I connected with her and thanked her for keeping a steady pace. She replied, "Not too bad, I'm 76 years old!"

We ran a good race and she was in excellent shape! She was so cool!

There's this quote from the video that I love! It's something that I do my best to live by every day:
Just keep pushing. it doesn't matter who is in front of you. There is no competition. Just do your best. What I'm looking forward to now, tonight, tomorrow and ongoing is to just do my very best. It's all I can do.

When we give it our best, we win. That's the most we can ask of ourselves. So, be kind, be patient, allow for setbacks, and keep going!

Assignment:
Think about a time when competition (or jealousy – that's okay!) inspired you to push yourself to reach a goal. The important thing here is that it moved you to action, despite what the influence is. If being angry about something inspired good action, that's fine because the *action* was good! Give yourself plenty of time to write about this and give details. You can write about multiple experiences, people, and/or situations that drove you to aim high and work toward a goal. This can be any type of goal – career, education, fitness and so on!

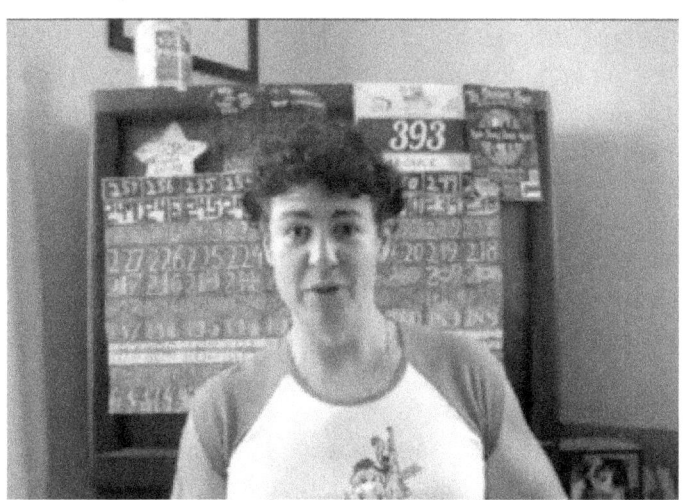

Reason #92 – <u>So I can be the best hunter that I can be</u>
Recorded on April 7, 2014

This was another reason inspired by <u>The Hunger Games</u>, and zombie fiction! The characters in those stories were able to provide for themselves because they were resourceful hunters, and that had a big influence on me. Plus, feeding people is one of my favorite activities! As a successful hunter, I'd have plenty of meat to share in meals and to give away!

I thought it would be cool to learn how to skillfully and compassionately hunt to eat organic, clean-fed, free-range animal proteins, and also to help control animal populations in overly dense areas. During certain times of the year, wildlife management seeks hunters to help control the animal population in specific areas to help maintain ecological balance. Some animals are not indigenous to an area, and are impacting the ecosystem adversely. Hunters help bring balance to these areas; there is a need for them! Instead of just kill these animals, responsible hunters use and consume the animal proteins. When done properly, hunting can be humane, compassionate and immensely beneficial to the environment!

I come from hunters and farmers. Growing up, my grandfather had an amazing, HUGE garden in his front yard, and my father would go

223

hunting during deer season. He wasn't very good at it, but he enjoyed it so much that he kept on going. I remember the first time he caught a deer and we had an enormous feast at my grandmother's house. We were all so proud of him, and most of all, he was proud of himself. That weekend, he took my sister and I to my grandparent's backyard and taught us how to shoot rifles and a bow. I wasn't very skilled at it, but I sure did enjoy it. It wasn't until years later that I went to a gun range and then an archery range. I'm still not very good (yet), and it's going to be an ongoing work in progress until I feel ready to go hunting with friends!

Activity:
If hunting is appealing to you, then your activity here is to research what you'd like to hunt, the season to do it, and what supplies you'll need (firearm, ammunition, traps, archery equipment, clothing, binoculars and such). Researching these things will help you see how much money, time and training you'll need to invest in this endeavor. It'll also help plant the seed in your mind to visualize it and bring it closer to reality.

If you'd prefer not to hunt (or if you'd like a bonus activity), then plan a garden – it can be as simple as a few herbs in a kitchen window. Do some research to see what you can do with the space you have. Then, start simply. Purchase potting soil, seeds, and get it going! Practice the same principle here that you do with your goals – start with some basics and build on slowly from there. Most importantly, just get started!

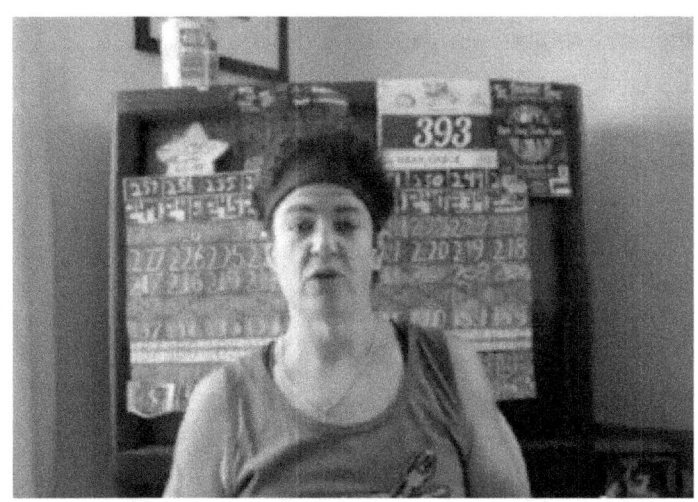

Reason #93 – <u>Because reaching this goal will motivate me to reach more</u>
Recorded on April 11, 2014
Weight: 167 pounds

Successful people use goals as stepping stones for growth, and never stop striving for personal development.

I really wish I could take full responsibility for the insights expressed here, and if I did, that would be letting my ego completely take over. Full disclosure here – I've had great influences, and I hope that you do as well. By speaking with people who have what I want, reading books, articles and blogs, my mind has an inventory that I can draw ideas from. By putting together pieces from various influences, I'm able to come up with solutions to a variety of problems. Additionally, the solutions for both the problem itself as well as how to utilize the habit of action are implemented.

The right time waits for no one; the present is the right time. There's no better time than now. There is no perfect scenario, we create it. Whether it's weight loss, getting up early, being disciplined about a financial budget, keeping anxiety at bay, staying clean and sober, or managing anger issues, it's all related to the same thing – the desire to make a change, taking action, and then creating and maintaining a habit.

Once we become successful at something, many of us realize that reaching a goal is great, but it was the journey that was the best part. It creates another habit – a habit of continually growing and striving for excellence. It's something that I've been inspired to do by the greatest influences I've found so far in business, personal development, life coaches, motivational speakers, authors, spiritual leaders, yoga teachers, amazing roller derby skaters, endurance race champions and sponsored athletes. These people are always working on *something*!

Successful people never stop growing! May we continue to rise to the occasion every time we embark on a goal, reach it, and then set our sights on the next!

An obligation of success is to share the experience. Actions speak louder than words, and our actions inspire others to follow their dreams, to figure out what their hearts truly want, and to go at it, full-speed! The first step in this process is to be that example, to inspire change by *being* the change. Once we've accomplished a huge goal, we can now show others how it's done!

Questions:
How does it feel when you've accomplished a goal?
What are your goals for the week?
How do you plan to reach those goals?

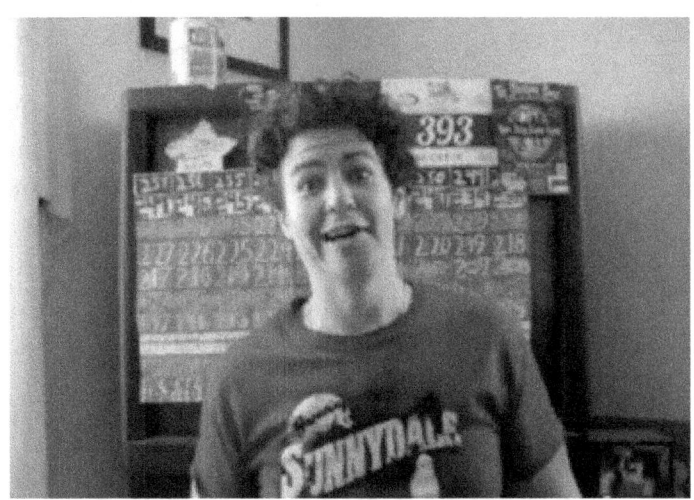

Reason #94 - <u>To improve my 5K times</u>
Recorded on April 19, 2014
Weight: 161 pounds

I've covered races in previous reasons, but this one pertains to 5K races. I was still hot and heavy on the idea of running races when I wrote my list. Again, I've lost the interest in running, but I still incorporate some of the training principles in my fitness routine.

A personal favorite is high intensity interval training! Circuit training has vastly improved my overall endurance and my speed on skates! Plus the challenge has expanded my mind in ways I hadn't conceived, thanks to pushing past my comfort zone and finding new potential that I otherwise would have not tapped into. It's just as much mental training as it is physical.

Fitness is a reward, not a punishment. Too often we force ourselves to do something because it's "healthy," and we want to burn fat, lose weight, work off a cheat meal and so on. If we use fitness as a punishment for bad actions, we eventually come to resent it. Then, we start finding reasons to skip a workout. Eventually, we go back to bad habits with food. See the pattern here?

When we work out, we should do something fun, engaging, motivating, and thrilling! Running for me had lost its appeal, and now my routine is a combination of cross-training which includes weight lifting, high intensity intervals, roller skating, various styles of yoga, dancing, cycling, and whatever else strikes my fancy! Mixing it up is great for my metabolism, my attention span, and my insatiable curiosity for new and challenging things!

This is an elaborate way of saying I replaced my resentment of running with things I like. It still can be a challenge, so again, the best way to prepare is to get started. Get dressed in workout clothes. Stretch. Warm up. Listen to awesome music. Get moving!

Challenge:
Set a realistic goal right now. It can be something on your list that you haven't embarked on just yet, or something you've been holding back on, or are intimidated by. Next, take that goal and multiply it by 10. Does it seem outlandish, scary, impossible? Good. It should be frightening. Fear is just inexperience; we fear what we don't understand. So, if your goal is to hold a 1-minute plank, get ready to hold a 10-minute plank. This doesn't mean that you have to hold it the whole time – take a breather when needed, and then come right back into it. Do you want to save $1000 to take a vacation? Imagine what you would and could do to save $10,000. Doesn't that sound WAY more exciting? Set a HUGE goal, meditate on it for at least 20 minutes, taking slow, deep, mindful breaths as you do so. Inhale deeply through your nose, filling your lungs, chest and the back of your throat to capacity. Hold that breath. Then, slower than the inhale, exhale it through your nose. As you meditate on your goal, practice this deep breathing, focusing on your breath and visualizing your goal. Once your 20 minutes are up, write down your thoughts. Express any fears you had coming into this, and how you feel about it now. Hold nothing back. Then, write down action items that you can take this month to work toward that goal. Next, break those down into weekly tasks. Then, write your weekly schedule, day by day. Finally, in one month, crush that goal! If anything, reaching for something way beyond our original goals gets us much further than we had originally anticipated! Journal

throughout the month, focusing on your goal, your actions, and anything that's getting in your way. Practice all the habits we've worked on leading to this point – be accountable, honest, and ready to take action! Most of all, enjoy the journey!

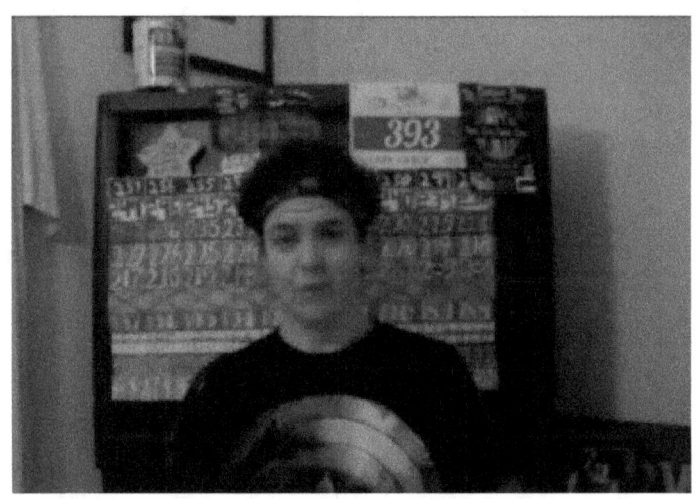

Reason #95 – <u>Because I love to earn things and this will take time</u>
Recorded on April 24, 2014
Weight: 161 pounds

Making a healthy lifestyle transition is so much more than just eating right, exercising and losing weight. It's about making a total shift in mind, body and spirit. It's a process, and as we embark on our goal, it's important to enjoy the steps in the journey. There's so much beauty in the subtle things, and when we focus on the end, we lose sight of the present.

Enjoy the process of earning something huge, and how this process creates our best life; it helps us become our greatest selves, and teaches us to live truly, passionately, and wholly authentically. Watch and marvel how things happen slowly, intricately, and subtly. It's beautiful.

Self-acceptance takes time. So often, we rely on others to validate us. We try to fit in. Over the course of time, hardships and our personal journey, we ultimately realize that the love we create for ourselves can *never* be taken away. We love ourselves for precisely who we are, as we are! It's a blessing to be unique and extraordinary! Anyone trying to assimilate will ultimately realize that there's NO pleasing people. There's no perfect formula, there's no perfect person.

There are over 7 billion of us, all composed of the same materials, but ultimately we are all unique. Pardon the corny reference here – stay with me though, because it works – but we're all like snowflakes in a blizzard. Each snowflake is made of the same exact materials, and yet they're all beautiful and unique. They're all a part of something bigger, and are both extraordinary by themselves, and beautiful when joined together.

Just like a snow storm, there is beauty, even though snow can be a royal pain in the ass. However, when we take a moment to observe how beautiful it is, how quiet things get, and the many fun things we can do in the snow, we can appreciate it. Snow provides good reason to snuggle up with someone, by a fire, drinking hot tea or cocoa from mugs, and stay warm together.

Just like a snow storm can bring us together, so can all of our commonalities. Once we can see past the things that annoy us (which, when we see them in others, are really reflections of things that annoy us about ourselves), then we can see the great qualities (again, a reflection of the things we see in others that we like about ourselves).

That's how it SHOULD be. We have much in common and we're ALL connected. That's a wonderful thing! We're extraordinarily diverse, and vastly beautiful in our uniqueness.

The ability to be ourselves, unabashedly, good-heartedly and well-intendedly embracing our unique scars, flaws and whole selves is a wonderful process that both creates AND changes our lives.

It creates our lives in the sense that it gives us freedom to be our true, authentic, fully integrated selves. I like to think of people (myself included) as mansions. Not just mere houses, but vast, huge and detailed mansions. When we accept ourselves fully, we allow every door in our expansive mansions to be wide open. We may not absolutely love everything that is in every room, but we accept that's just part of our mansion. We may see our healthy habits like the gardens and grass on our property – it's something that adds value, and the better we maintain it, the more value it creates.

A lifestyle change takes time. It's a process, and it's definitely worth the time and effort to do it. At first, it requires willpower. Willpower is the initial burst to help us make small shifts and changes in our routine to take action on a new habit. Repetition of the action establishes the habit. Then, that habit creates lasting, sustainable change. It's hard to get started, and it gets to become a routine the more we do it. It's not always easy, and it may never be easy, but it creates lasting change that is definitely worth it!

Without our flaws, we'd have very little reason to work on personal development. These perceived shortcomings, or flaws, are actually an amazing part of our character, and the changes we create in our lives serve as an amazing life lesson. The change is for the better, because it helps us realize our flaws are just as fabulous as our assets!

It takes time and a lot of work, mistakes and humility to accept ourselves, own up to our defects, and learn to love every facet of our being. It happens, though. It will. And when it does, it's monumental!

Activity:
Set a date and get together with a group. Invite everyone to write down some huge life goals. Encourage them to aim high, to be ambitious, and to make it something they've *always* wanted to do (a BIG one for me was skydiving – and it was life-changing when I actually did it!). Then, have everyone place their goals into a bowl in the center of a table (or wherever you are gathering). One by one, have them draw out a written goal (if they get their own goal, have them draw a different one). Once everyone has another person's goal, have everyone write action items, suggestions and advice to help reach that goal. Have them help create a time line, a budget (if needed), and how they'll help the goal's creator along the way.

It's always easier to give other people advice because we're less emotionally involved in their issues than we are in our own. This activity is designed to get input to help reach goals and to share the experience with others.

Feel free to have multiple goals, and to create a goal-bowl monthly gathering!

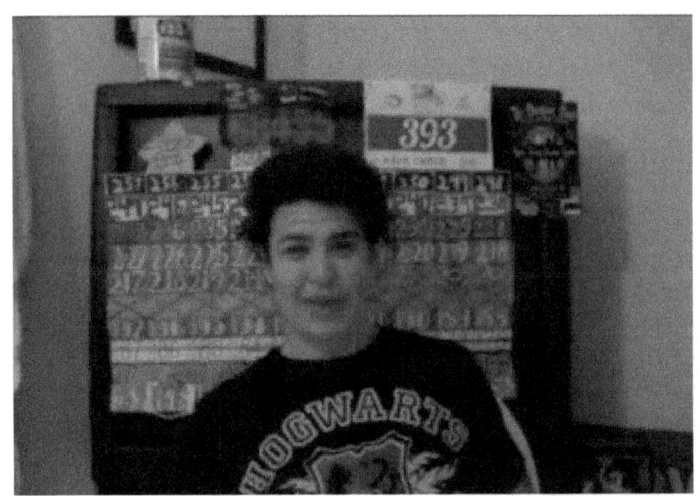

Reason #96 – <u>Because back fat is annoying when I sit down</u>
Recorded on May 5, 2014
Weight: 166 pounds

Excess fat makes it difficult for our bodies to work optimally. We need a healthy spine to support our bodies properly, and if we sit a lot while carrying excess fat, it makes it even harder for the spine to do its job. Without ample core strength, our spines fall victim to gravity, and over time, form into a shape that is not conducive for proper posture and physical health.

Back fat is unappealing, and is also bad for my back issues. Losing excess fat has certainly helped relieve the pain I've experienced for years, and eating clean has helped immensely!

From the video for this reason:
I remember when I would sit and I would feel a physical bulge behind me as soon as my ass hit the chair…and it was my back fat. It really serves me no purpose aesthetically or functionally.

Our bodies function in a very mechanical, scientific manner, and as we fuel ourselves with what our bodies need (not what our egos want) and stay active, our bodies reciprocate in kind.

There is a natural equilibrium that occurs when we put the right things into our bodies, and move them the ways that they've been designed to move. When we get out of whack (very technical term here), there's usually a cause to it. While factors like genetics and accidents are beyond our control, there are plenty of things that are within our control.

For instance, we can't change where we come from, we can't re-code our genetics and we can't do much to change how we were raised. We're born into the bodies we have, just like we were born into the houses we were raised in. However, our houses and our bodies are subject to ongoing maintenance, repairs, and upgrades. Our backs are very much like the foundation of a house – if we take good care of it, what we build on top is fortified by that solid foundation. By taking good care of our backs (and keeping off excessive back fat), our bodies will function optimally. Staying fit, eating healthy foods and maintaining good posture are several ways that we can keep our backs strong! A good back serves our entire bodies favorably!

Now that I have less fat on my back (and my body as a whole), there is a remarkable difference when I sit down, when I work out, when I drive, and when I do ordinary, everyday things. Standing, washing the dishes, even going to the bathroom used to be a challenge because my body was taxed by the extra weight on my back. It affected my posture and made me lean forward. I would hunch my shoulders, which made my chest tight. Leaning forward affected my neck and my entire upper back, which caused alignment issues in my spine.

Years of toting around excess fat on my back, coupled with my injuries, has affected my spine permanently, which is why it is so important for me to stay fit, and to practice daily good habits to keep my back in alignment. Some of the most beneficial daily practices I utilize are good nutrition (to keep the fat off), practicing yoga (to keep balance in my body, mind and spirit), and working my core muscles to keep good posture. These habits have improved my life remarkably! Also, on an aesthetic note, I LOVE how good my back looks! My back is actually the main image on the blog section of my website!

235

Questions:

Do you ever feel uncomfortable doing everyday things (such as sitting, driving and such)?

What do you think it would be like to feel comfortable doing these things?

How do you see the solution to this?

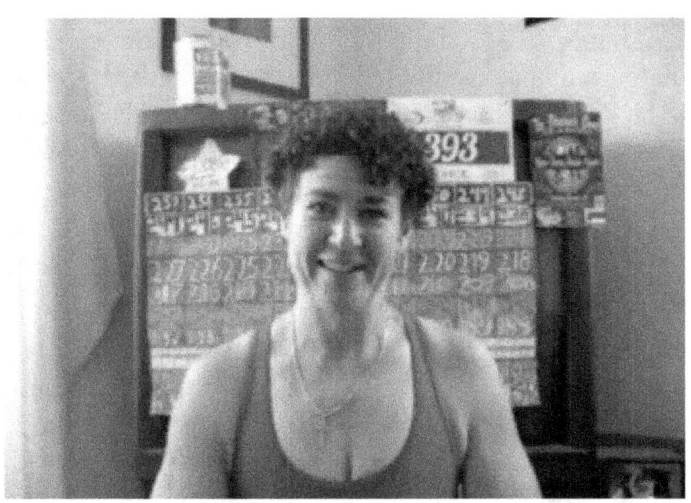

Reason #97 – <u>To one day climb up poles, gates and barriers in theme park lines</u>
Recorded on May 9, 2014
Weight: 159 pounds

I don't know why I've always had this inclination, but whenever I've waited in a queue for a theme park ride – roller coasters, log flumes, bumper cars and such – I wanted to scale walls and go all Spiderman on things. Every time I've been in a line that has barriers, walls, stairs, and gates, I've imagined jumping all the way up. It's not even for the sake of getting in front of the line, it would just be for the sake of being a wall-scaling bad ass!

The fantasy of it is more appealing than the actual action of it, as I learned in rock wall climbing!

After I'd gone rock climbing, I found out I wasn't particularly fond of it. Perhaps with time and more experience, I'll grow to like it more. Admittedly, my first and only attempt was after I had a huge setback. My rock climbing experience was a friend's remedy for recovering from a harrowing ordeal— The setback I mentioned earlier. I became obsessed with a woman. Following *really* bad advice, I drove over 800 miles from Florida to Maryland in a day to tell that woman that I had deep feelings for her. I was rejected.

Right after it happened, I called my friend in Washington, D.C., told her what happened, and she invited me over. We talked, we laughed, I cried, and the healing process began. Then, the next day, she took me rock climbing.

The rock wall got me to face some deep-seeded issues and fears – that, after all this time and work investing in myself, I still had *more* work to do. I was still relying on others to validate me. That drive to Maryland and everything leading up to it – thinking, daydreaming, fantasizing, having conversations (real and imagined) and ultimately mourning a woman I had become obsessed with – robbed me of time that I could have otherwise spent on investing in *myself*. My obsession with that woman, and the actions I took, caused me to do the very SAME things I had done in the past with food, alcohol, drugs, and money. I was still trying to fill a void in a *very* unhealthy way.

I had to confront and deal with these issues. It all happened on that rock wall.

I hated it...at first. My mind kept focusing on the rejection from the previous day. I couldn't see myself succeeding. All I saw was failure. So, I kept falling off. It sucked so badly. When I say it sucked, I mean it really, really sucked. My palms were sweaty, my heart was racing, my chest was tight, and I felt like such a poor-me, sad story loser. I couldn't get out of my head.

Eventually, I was able to scale one of the walls. My friend invited me to join her again...and I'm going to do it.

Life never gives us a straightforward path. For me, I always find that when things are going well, life reminds me that it's never going to be easy, but if I stay true to myself, surround myself with encouraging, intelligent, and take-no-bullshit friends, I'll get through whatever comes my way, one wall at a time.

Assignment:
Imagine having a super power – pick one or several! Write about what you would do with it, and why you want this power. It can be anything from a physical power (like super strength, healing abilities, and flying), to a mental ability (mind-reading, mind control), or a special skill (having a Midas touch, having the power to reach into your pocket and always have the exact amount of money to get something you need or want). Get creative! Write about this for at least 20 minutes, going as long as you'd like to. Focus on what you'd have, what you'd do, and why you'd do these amazing things. Elaborate on why you want that super power, and the why it is significant for you.

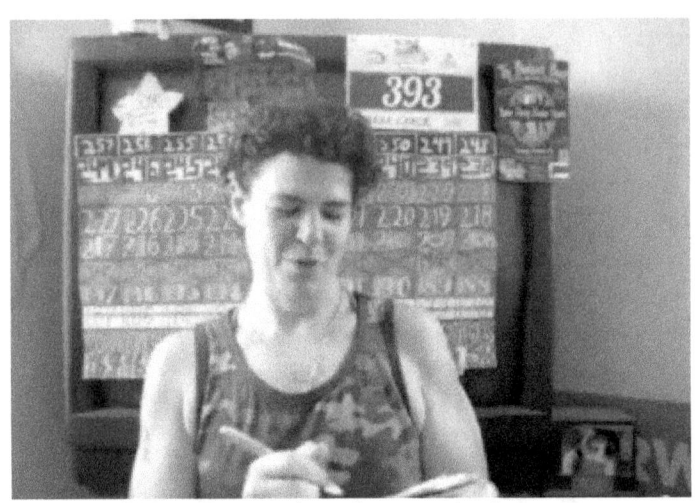

Reason #98 – <u>So my ring size won't change anymore</u>
Recorded on May 26, 2014
Weight: 159 pounds

This reason pertains to ring size, and what I really was getting to was marriage. Since marriage is supposed to be a lifelong commitment, I want my ring size to stay the same. Just as I want my ring size to stay the same, I want to keep healthy habits in mind, body and spirit for myself and for whomever I spend the rest of my life with, when the time comes. The same things I want for myself are the same things I'd want for my wife – happiness, health, abundance and a life filled with shared love.

Loving myself makes me available for real, true, sincere love. Loving myself keeps my love tank full, so I can continue to spread it around. Loving myself means I can openly share with others, keeping that which I have by giving it away. When we love ourselves, that wellspring is self-sustaining.

For me, self-love comes from recognizing there is a greater good. There is something that dances with me in this life that keeps my energy high and my engine going. It's not food, it's not drugs, it's not booze and it's not sex; it's so much more profound than any of those. It never runs out, it never gives up, it never goes away. It's everlasting and indestructible.

It is a part *of* us, not apart *from* us. We all have access to it and we all share it. Whatever name we call it, it's the great driving force that inspires us to spread Light out into this world and let it into our hearts and minds. Tapping into it is a conscious choice, and once we make that choice (and let go of our ego), we can find that source of good.

Personally, I call that force God. To me, God is Good without the redundant "O" – God doesn't need the extra O, He's omnipotent!

I look forward to the day when I find the one who can love, appreciate, and see that amazing light in me, own it within herself, and to share it with me for a lifetime. When I do, I'm putting a ring on her finger, and I shall wear mine proudly!

Activity:
Write a letter to yourself from five years into the future. Imagine you've reached a huge milestone and several more. In this letter, let your future self give your current self encouragement, sharing insight, thoughts, feelings, and the experience of what it's like to have something that you've wanted and worked for. Once you've completed the letter, add it to your notebook or on your board from Reason #5, and read the letter at least once a week.

See what we're doing here? We're turning out thoughts into objectives, and setting our minds up to receive! The practice of *believing* comes from *doing*.

I sure hope you're doing these assignments – they've worked for me! So far, I've achieved everything I've set out to do. That's no exaggeration – I mean *everything*. There's a reason for that. Hope is the only thing stronger than fear. It fuels the drive to be successful. Practice hope, faith, and dreaming – do the assignments and write about the experiences! You'll amaze yourself with your capabilities!

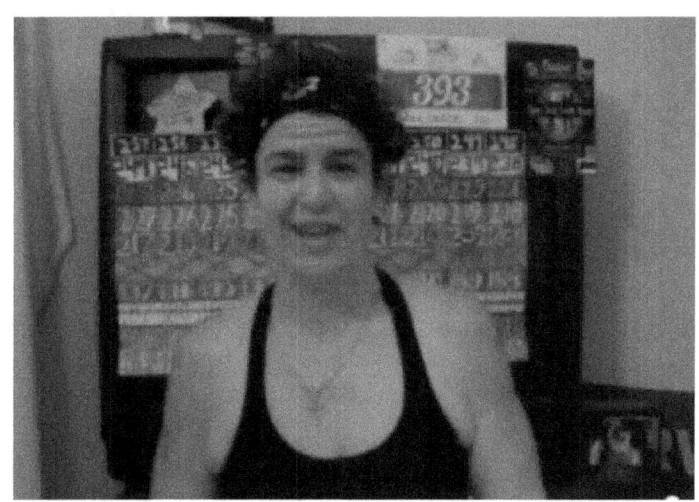

Reason #99 – <u>To quit bitching and keep living</u>
Recorded on May 27, 2014

From the video for this reason:
This ain't just about me, it's about trying to save people's lives! It's about trying to make people happy! I can't do that for you; you can do it for yourself. I'm going through the motions, and this is my journey. I'm hoping to plant the seeds so that when you're ready, you do it. When will you be ready? Only you will know. Come back to this and remember that you CAN do it. Anybody is capable of doing it if you commit to it, prepare for it, and change the way you think and change your habits. THAT is what changes your actions. NOW. Right NOW. Today is your Monday. How badly do you want it? Do you want to do it? I know I wanted it badly! I ain't even weighed in yet and I'm almost two pounds from my goal. Have you seen the series? Have you heard me talk about the fact that I had been obese for twenty years? I've never EVER been a fit adult, ever. It took me over two years to get to this point and the whole journey started EIGHT years ago. A lifetime! But, it just happens when you choose it to happen. Work, family, finances...bullshit. That's all noise. You will find a way, or you will be a victim of your excuses. It all comes down to choice. What do you want to choose to do? I choose to live the rest of my life healthy. It starts now, and today. One day at a time. Stick with me. This isn't the

end of it. This is just the beginning. And I believe in you. From my heart to yours, I believe in you.

Complaining achieves nothing productive. It feeds the ego, makes us victims, drops our energy, and keeps us doing the same repetitive things, giving us the same repetitive results.

What does it take to be successful? Actions—it takes the courage to try. So, just *try*. Keep trying until you get good at it, and then keep going. It just takes one step, then another, and then another. They happen one at a time, and every small step leads to huge progress over time. It just happens, little by little, and then it all comes together. We progress, we take steps back, and we rise again and keep on moving. The only way we get stronger is by getting up every time we fall. When we rise from a fall, it establishes a mindset that we CAN do something. It may take a while, and we may have to do it a LOT of times to get it right, but it happens with effort. It happens in small, everyday increments. It's gradual, and it's humbling.

It creates victors, Smashing Success Stories, and champions.

Pursuing a dream, working toward a goal, and doing something life-changing is what makes the difference between existing and *living*. So, do that! LIVE! Go for it!

You can do it! I believe in you!

Challenge:
Go an entire day without any complaints. If you feel one rising, express something you're grateful for, something you're happy about, or what you want to do about the thing you're itching to bitch about. Update your journal at the end of the day. Once you've had a successful day, plan to do it another day. Then, once you've had at least two successful, continuous complaint-free days, do it for a week. Then, keep going.

See how far you can go, and journal throughout your experience.

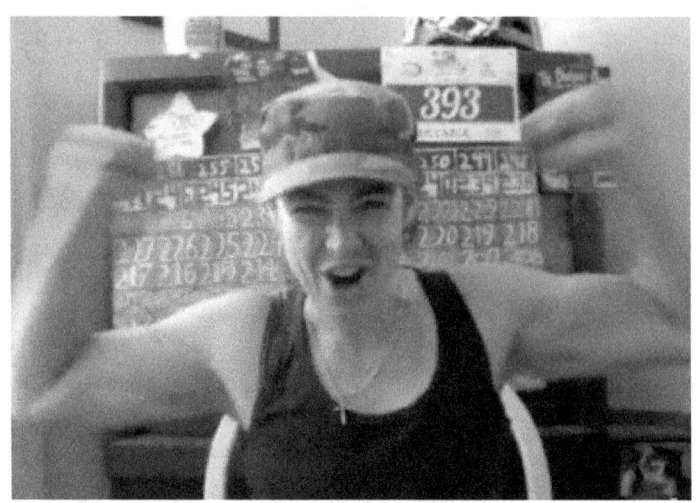

Reason #100 – <u>For a fresh start</u>
Recorded on July 14, 2014
Weight: 156 pounds

Reason 100...I DID IT!!! Those last three pounds, my goodness were they stubborn pounds to lose. I would love to say that it was because of metabolism, a plateau, that my body was doing blah blah blah, but in all truth, I was having a bit of a personal issue with allowing myself success. All that hard work, all the time invested and all the amazing realizations that I had, and I was *still* struggling with allowing myself to have what I wanted and had worked SO hard for. Even sharing that truth is hard.

Something clicked in the beginning of July. Between May and July, my weeks were following this pattern: great Monday, solid Tuesday, pretty good Wednesday, a cheat meal and otherwise good Thursday...

...Then cheat meals Friday, Saturday and Sunday.

Some weeks there were one meal per day on those days, and the others were cheat days.

It took a couple months to finally commit to following through and hitting my goal, and on Tuesday, July 14, 2014, I got on the scale and weighed in at 156 pounds.

I DID IT! I lost 100 pounds! Well, even better, I lost 101, which pleased me to NO end, because I surpassed my goal AND 101 is a palindrome! Who doesn't love palindromes?!

As far as my excitement goes, I'll just share exactly what I shared in the video for Reason 100 - The video says it all!

July 14, 2014 should be known as the day I hit my GOAL!

I weighed in today at 156.2, BOOM! Which means I've lost 101 pounds. 100 pounds are GONE.

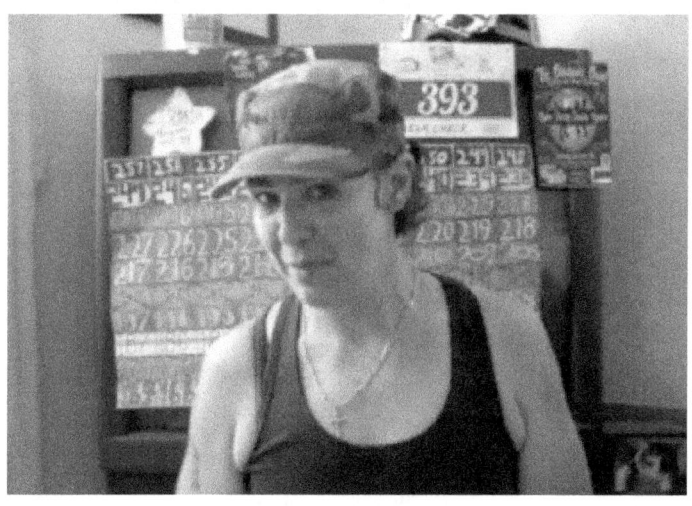

I'm realizing now that I have a hundredth reason, so I have to find my notebook to find the hundredth reason…it's been a minute since I've had to pull out this notebook…

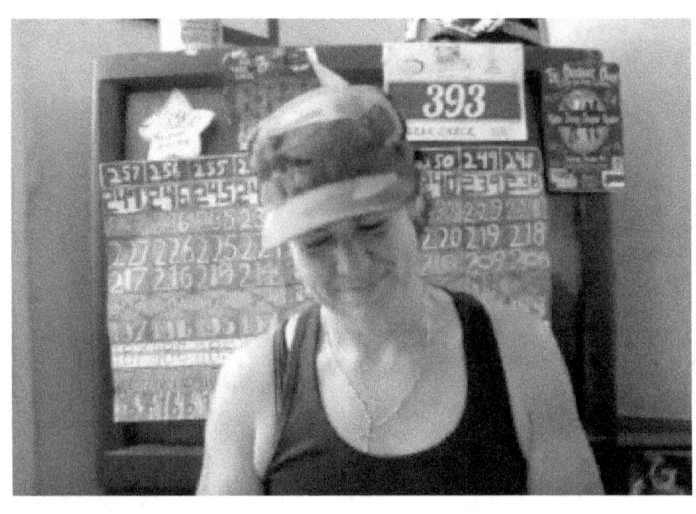

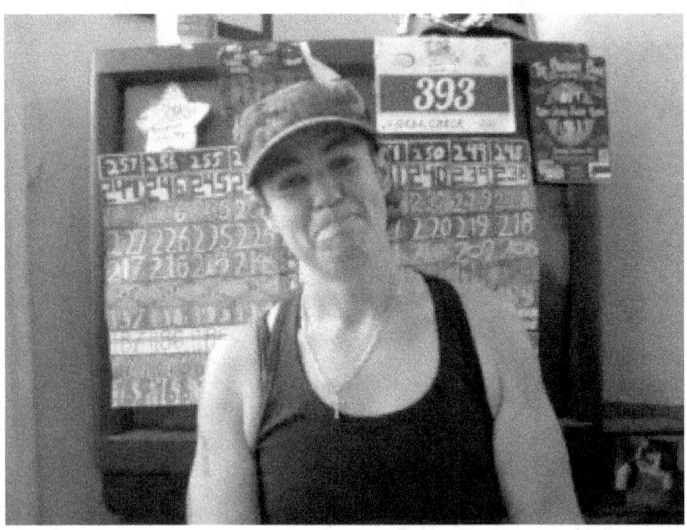

The hundredth reason on my list of 100 Reasons to Lose 100 Pounds is for a fresh start.

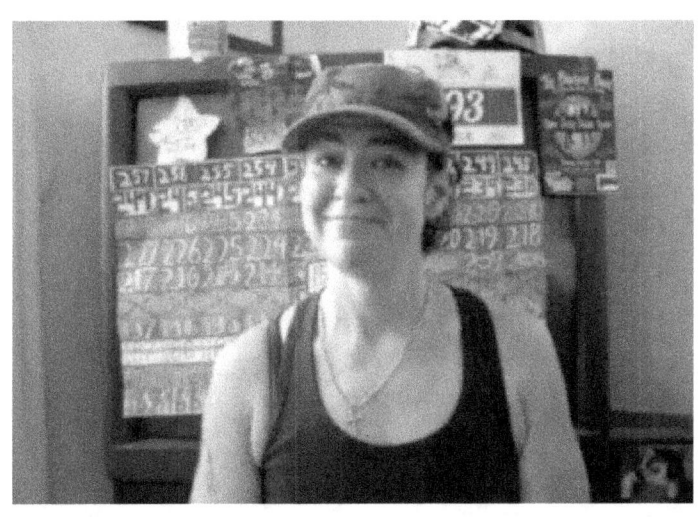

I have been praying for a clean slate for several years. Hitting my goal weight means that I'm going to live a healthy lifestyle for the rest of my life. I have more goals that I want to aim for. I want to keep toning up and I want to get shredded, but mostly, I just want to be fit for life and be healthy from now on. The past is in the past. This is my future; this is what I want to do with my life.

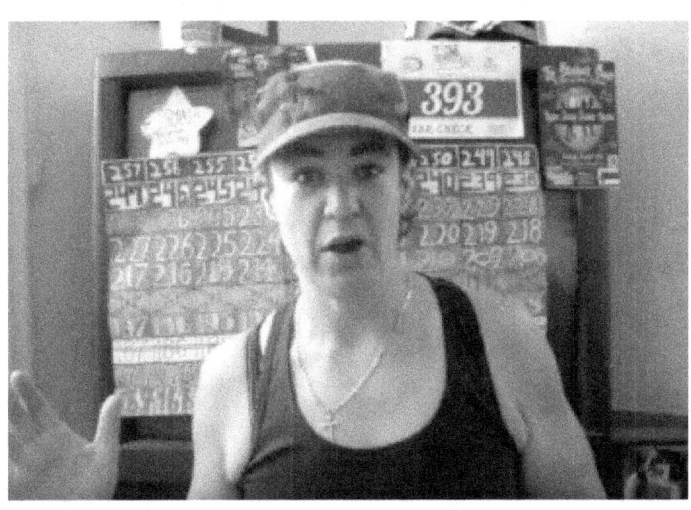

When I started this 101 pounds ago, I had a wish, I had a desire. I really had no idea that I could pull it off. And here we are. It took me

over two years, and there have been so many ups and downs. But, this is it. This is just the beginning. I'm going to continue to pursue excellence, and train like a champion, and work my ASS off, because I've earned it. I want to keep it, and tend to it, be smart with it and continue to make good decisions. I'm so excited about my future, about this project, and for what's going to happen. I will continue keeping an account of my journey, and there is so much more to come.

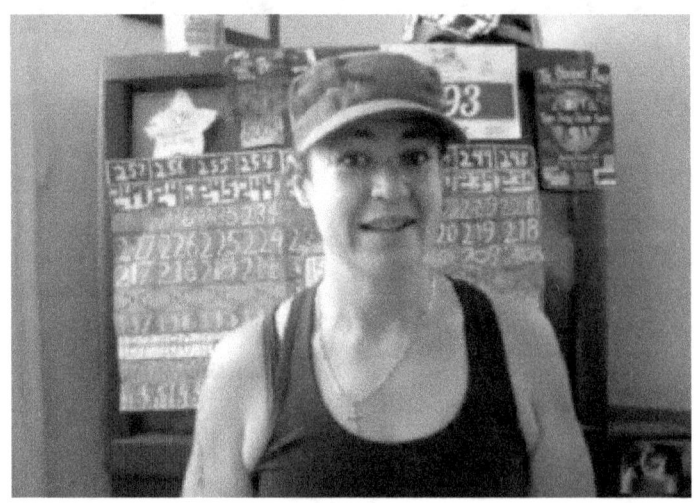

A clean slate. I have got the best starting point ever. My life starts right now.

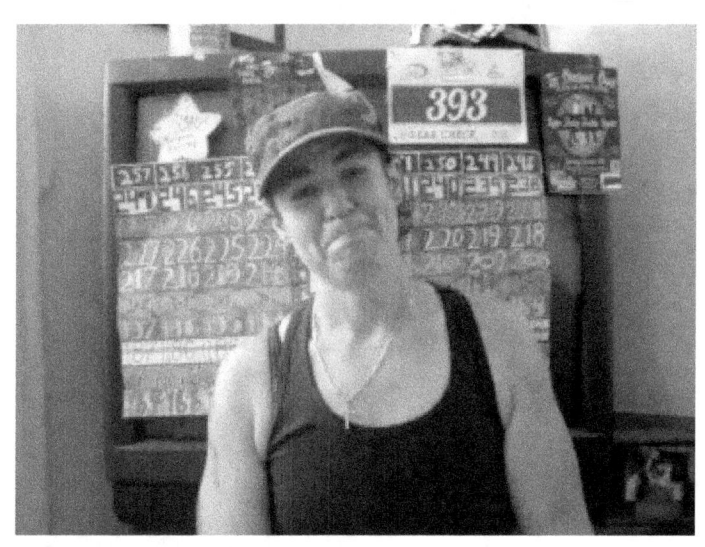

Thank you for being a part of this journey!

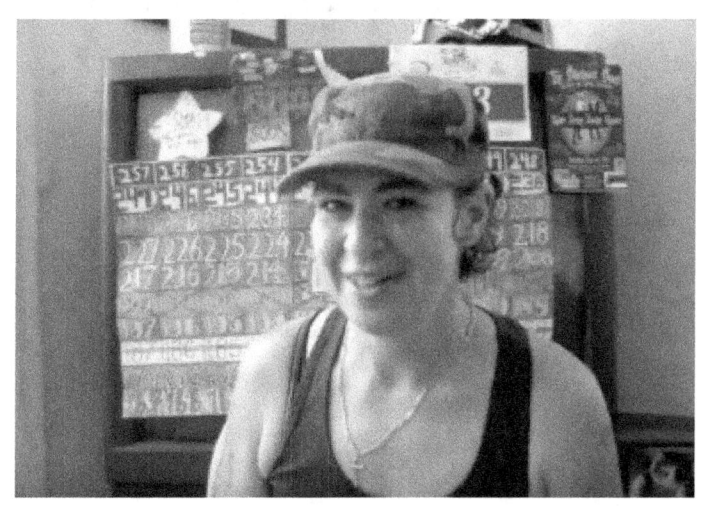

It's about to get SO much better.

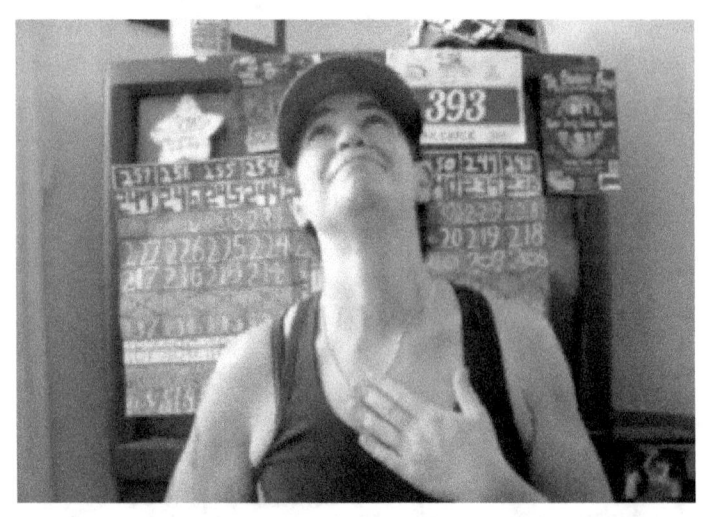

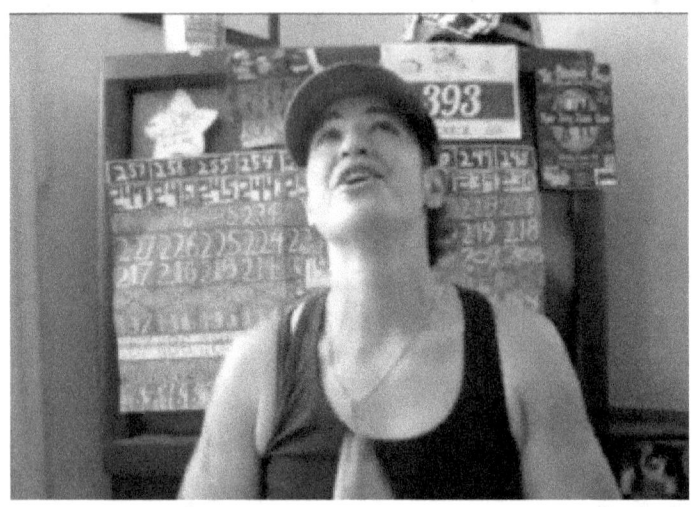

Thank you, God!

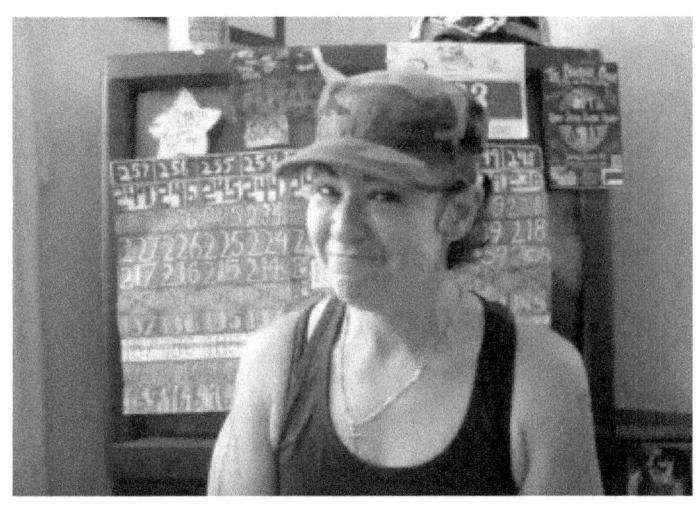

Here we go! I get to be fit for life! How lucky am I? It's amazing.

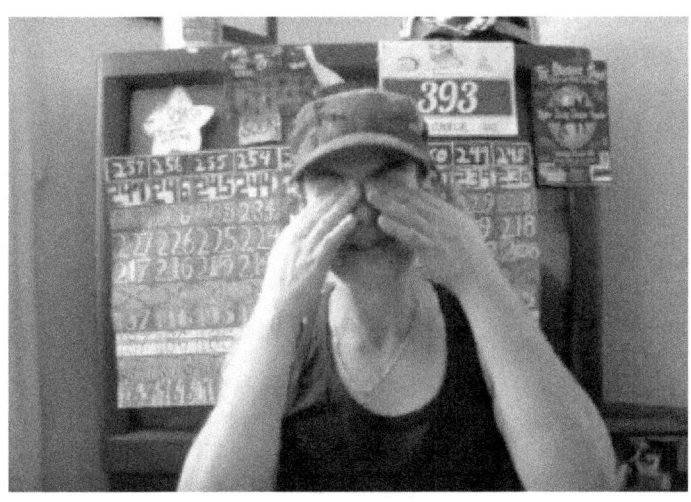

These are good.

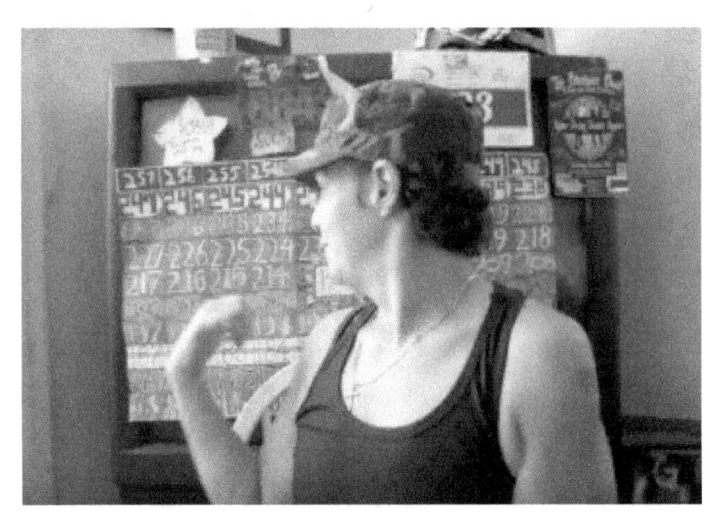

I wish you only the best. It can be done.

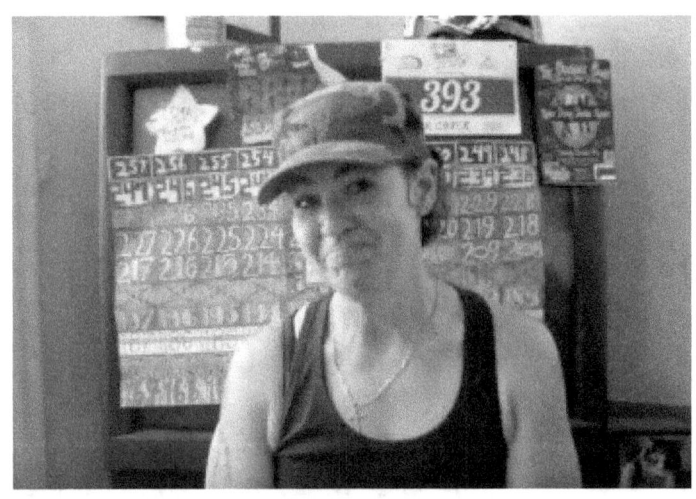

It CAN be done.

Assignment:

Keep writing in your journal. Document your endeavors. Gather with friends and family regularly. Look at your goals daily, and update them weekly. Refresh and review them every 6 months. Celebrate milestones. Recover from setbacks. Continue daily prayer and mindfulness practices. Stay close to loving, supportive, positive influences. Eat healthy, allowing room for indulgences in moderation. Plan a fitness routine and stick with it. Practice great habits in mind, body and spirit. Have lots of fun, soul-charging, mind-blowing, physically-challenging and mentally rewarding experiences. Serve others in your community. Seek wise counsel. Set outlandish goals and smash them. Share your light and love with others, without creating any attachment to an outcome. Give from the heart. Dance, sing, and laugh often. Get help when needed. Listen to your heart.

Live a full and abundant life, here and now!

Be your own hero!

Love yourself and share your love with the world!

Afterword

It's been over a year since I smashed my goal! Life has taken some amazing turns, and there certainly have been many ups and downs! When this all started, I really thought that losing 100 pounds and getting fit would fix my life. I thought that would be my happy ending.

Just like I stated in the last reason, it was just the beginning.

So many things happened in so many unpredictable ways, and as I remind my students and clients, we have no control over the tide. We can only control our rudder, and keep moving along.

I knew I was going to share my experience to encourage people, and as my life coach tells me, I'm responsible for the *what*— the *how* will reveal itself.

One of the many *how* components for maintaining my wellness and staying accountable is by leading my Army of 100. We are a group of goal-Smashing, success-oriented, cooperative and encouraging folks that are always looking to rise to the next level physically, mentally and spiritually.

The best way to move forward is with powerful people! People who work together thrive together, and it's my dream to see a healthy, happy, prosperous and peaceful world. Imagine if everyone could find bliss, love and abundance in our everyday lives? It would be paradise!

To make that happen in our world, we should surround ourselves with like-minded people. I'm always recruiting for the Army of 100. I'm thrilled to show people the road to success, and love to provide help and resources along the way.

Sound good? AWESOME!

Join us!

Here's how you can get started today:
http://mindheartswole.com/armyof100/

Also, here are my social networking pages:
Body and Swole on Facebook:
https://www.facebook.com/bodyandswole
Instagram: https://www.instagram.com/kpsmash/

There are also lots of resources for motivation, inspiration, fitness and nutrition on my website: http://mindheartswole.com/

It takes a great deal of courage to get started on any lifestyle change, and you are doing a brave and wonderful thing for yourself by taking the time to read this book! Thank you for giving me the opportunity to share my story, and I hope it gets you fired up to write your own!

I look forward to witnessing your amazing transformation – I say this with full confidence that you CAN do it, and when you are ready, you WILL do it! You are amazing just as you are, here and now, in all of your glory. Whatever treasures that are waiting to be excavated are ready and waiting for you to find them. They are with you always, inside of you and a part of you. When you're ready, it's time dig them out, bring them to the surface, and let them SHINE!

Here's to your success, and to sharing our light with the world around us, illuminating the path with strength and hope after we've risen from the darkness!

I wish you the greatest life ahead, filled with joy, laughter, abundance and love. Most of all, may you see that these gifts are always inside of you.

Looking forward to seeing you in the Army of 100!

All my best,

Karen Petersen, Smash Tank
Fearless Leader of the Army of 100
Smashing Success Story